The Paralysed Patient

The Paralysed Patient

ROBERT ROAF

MA, BCh, MChOrth, FRCS, FRCSE,

LRCP, DObstetRCOG

Professor of Orthopaedic Surgery
University of Liverpool
Consultant Orthopaedic Surgeon to the
United Liverpool Hospitals and
The Robert Jones and
Agnes Hunt Orthopaedic Hospital
Oswestry, Shropshire

and

LEONARD J. HODKINSON

SRN, RNT, ONC, FRSH

Regional Nurse
(Professional Education and Development)
Northern Regional Health Authority

BLACKWELL

SCIENTIFIC PUBLICATIONS

OXFORD LONDON EDINBURGH

MELBOURNE

©1977 Blackwell Scientific Publications
Osney Mead, Oxford, OX2 OEL
8 John Street, London, WC1N 2HY
9 Forrest Road, Edinburgh, EH1 2QH
P.O. Box 9, North Balwyn, Victoria, Australia

Roaf, Robert
    The paralysed patient.
    Bibl. – Index.
    ISBN 0 632 09470 2
    1. Title 2. Hodkinson, Leonard John
    616.8'42   RC 400
    Paralysis

First published 1977

Distributed in the
United States of America by
J. B. Lippincott Company Philadelphia,
and in Canada by
J. B. Lippincott Company of
Canada Ltd, Toronto

Filmset in Ireland by
Doyle Photosetting Limited, Tullamore
printed in Great Britain at
the Alden Press, Oxford
and bound by
Kemp Hall Bindery, Oxford

Contents

1 : The Problems of the Paralysed Patient

Definition of paralysis

Paralysis may be defined as the temporary or permanent loss of function in a living part. This can mean either the loss of sensation or of voluntary motion. Literally, paralysis means 'loosening from beside' and implying any motor or sensory disability.

Any voluntary movement (i.e., under conscious control) requires integrity of at least two motor neurones making a continuous pathway from the cortex of the cerebrum of the brain to the anterior grey horn of the spinal cord (see Fig. 1.1) and thence from the spinal cord down the limb (or other part) to the muscle (see Fig. 1.2). If any part of the pathway is destroyed or interrupted the stimulus passing to the muscles is lost or severely deranged.

If an upper motor neurone in the pathway from the cortex to the anterior horn cells is destroyed the affected muscles will be hypertonic and will contract in a peculiar 'cogwheel' fashion. The muscles do not waste away or atrophy; this is called 'spasticity' or spastic paralysis.

If, on the other hand, the neurone which forms the pathway between the spinal cord and the muscle is damaged, the muscle loses tone, withers away and the part becomes flail; this is called 'flaccidity' or flaccid paralysis.

There are also forms of paralysis which are due to psychological inhibition of motor activity in a part.

It is difficult for fit and healthy people to imagine the problems of the disabled. Daily living procedures which are simple to those who are well present major problems to the paralysed. Self testing applied to a daily routine of dressing, feeding or attending to the personal toilet demonstrates how much longer it takes to put on trousers or briefs when the back cannot be bent, or to pull on a sock when the knee or hip cannot be flexed, or to shave or apply cosmetics when the elbow cannot be fully used or small objects cannot be grasped.

These experiments demonstrate the lesser frustrations of the paralysed person. Many others, some far more important, recur all day and every day. Paralysis brings frustration in speed, movement and precision, in work as well as in leisure, in the static postures as well as in locomotion.

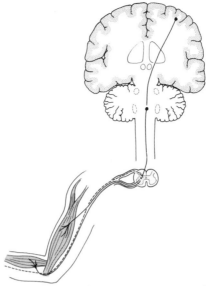

Fig. 1.1   The pathway from the cerebral cortex to the anterior grey horn of the spinal cord, down the spinal cord to the limb.

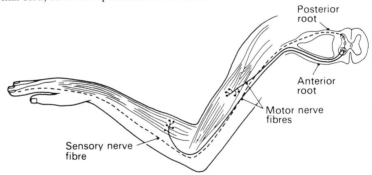

Fig. 1.2.   The nerve tract from the spinal cord to the muscle.

The impairment of muscular control of joints, limbs or the trunk in paralysis can cause flail limbs to flap about like the empty sleeves of a coat; or the limbs become stiff and jerky (cogwheel paralysis) so that movement is rough and uneven. They may shake and tremble at varying speeds so that precise delicate movements are impossible. These examples of paralysis prevent the performance of normal movements.

Adaptation to living with paralysis

Many paralysed people consider themselves normal because they lead a life which is full and vigorous despite their disability. They have developed 'trick' movements which enable them to do tasks which are performed differently by 'normal' people. Their movements may be slower and more cumbersome or maybe they may use some device to enable them to do a task. They may become exhausted achieving what they set out to do.

The adaptation to living a full life in the presence of a severe permanent disability depends upon many factors:

A desire for independence

The desire for financial or physical independence may be reflected by the need to be alone or a reluctance to rely upon social welfare funds or gifts from friends, relatives or philanthropic organizations. Thus, the disabled person often develops a method of personal care and of locomotion to satisfy his need for independence. He will learn a means of earning money, no matter how little, seeking the assistance of a sympathetic employer who will allow him to work from a wheelchair or crutches. Earning capacity, craftsmanship and independence from sources of charitable or social welfare funds contribute to self respect and personal satisfaction.

A desire for security

A welfare state which cares for the sick and disabled usually supplies adequate funds for the support of the family of the disabled breadwinner. However, some countries do not give such aid and a total absence of income makes it necessary for a paralysed person to find a means of earning. The strong instinct to care for our dependents often overcomes severe obstacles.

A desire for affection

Permanent paralysis and severe disability may make normal social inter-relationship difficult. Limitation of locomotion often confines the paralysed person and makes excursions infrequent. For the disabled, each venture out of the house may require the detailed planning of route and equipment that others would make for an expedition to an unexplored region of the world. Choice of hotel for a holiday necessitates correspondence to find out if there are lifts, if the toilet is adjacent to the bedroom or if the dining room and doors are large enough for a wheelchair. There are many examples of the complexity of living which limits the disabled person's opportunities for meeting people outside the usual circle of relatives or attendants.

These limitations tend to make a confined patient into a lonely intro-

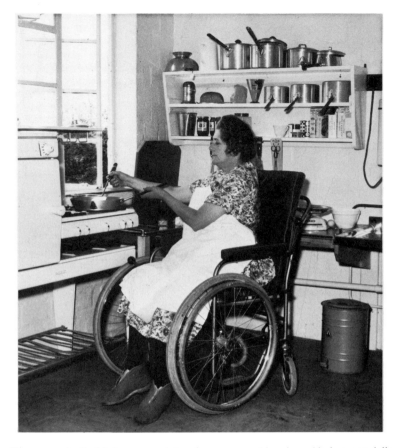

Fig. 1.3. A disabled woman doing her own cooking in a kitchen specially designed for her.

vert. The disability may itself lead to a personality defect: the individual may be shy, awkward and limited in range and topics of conversation. Repetitive conversation with the dedicated attendants may lead to frustration, which may be concealed or demonstrated in irritability and temper.

The paralysed-disabled person requires love, affection and contact with others as do all people. Unfortunately his physical condition makes him less likely to satisfy such needs. Organizations (many of them run by volunteers) which cater for the social needs of people with disabilities are a great help. There is a danger, however, that those who need help most are the ones who reject it for physical or emotional reasons or through pride and a dislike of receiving charity.

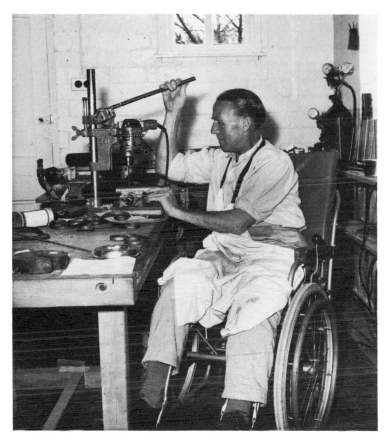

Fig. 1.4. A disabled man able to carry out his trade in a specially designed workshop.

The desire for change

Disability, as mentioned may lead to loneliness because of limitation of locomotion and confinement to a small area. All of us enjoy a break from routine. A different menu, a change of working hours, new clothes, a visit to a cinema, a holiday or a trip abroad are part of the necessary release from tension and contribute to psychological balance.

The problem of pain

Pain is a necessary evil. It is the mechanism that reports that all is not well in a part of the body. Without pain we would not know that a limb or organ was hurt or infected and in need of protection and treatment. For example, absence of pain and sensation in a joint (due to a nervous disorder, called a neuropathy) can cause a patient to continue to abuse a hurt joint.

Usually pain is of a temporary nature and can be relieved with treatment. Often the remedy is one we can apply ourselves, or may require moderate medical or dental treatment.

Pain in some patients, however, may be excruciating or mild, but nagging and unrelieved by common remedies. The worst type of pain is knowing that it will not go away and prevents sleep.

The toleration of pain varies; one individual will exaggerate complaints of a mild pain while another will play down complaints of a severe pain. Many factors can cause these variations—temperament, emotional state and general health all play a part. Nurses, however, must never ignore complaints of pain. They may be significant and must always be reported to the doctor in charge. The report may contribute to the diagnosis. Continuous unrelieved pain can contribute to the deterioration of a patient. Many drugs are available to control this.

The problem of obesity

Food is required by the body for many purposes; one of these is the production of energy to enable the body to work and perform exercise. Some disabled people are extremely limited in the amount of exercise and work they can do. Therefore, there is a danger that reserves of nutrition, taken in a diet, may be deposited as fat in the body with subsequent increase in weight. People who are confined to bed or wheelchairs for much of their time must restrict their diet to prevent this. Their appetite is often physiologically poor anyway.

The problem of a suitable dwelling

The ability to stand, walk and climb stairs without applying much thought to what we are doing, means that we can choose our own place to dwell and our own manner of living. This freedom of choice is often denied a person who is seriously disabled.

If locomotion depends upon a wheelchair, the house which the person occupies must have wide doors, a hallway without awkward angles and a ground-floor lavatory designed to allow the wheelchair to be positioned correctly. Devices such as hoists may also be installed to enable the person to move from the chair. If no suitable lift is available the disabled chairbound person must stay on the ground floor (a bungalow may be a sensible better choice if any choice is possible). Steps and stairs are a severe obstacle to many physically handicapped people even though they are not chairbound.

The problem of shopping

Towns, cities and all forms of public transport were devised for the fit person who can negotiate steps and stairways quickly and efficiently, open plateglass swing doors or revolving doors, sit on a stool at a snack bar counter, or enter the narrow rows of chairs in a cinema or theatre. Each of these movements is difficult for a person who is disabled or who is slowed up through ageing. Even carrying a walking stick complicates daily living; how do you cope with a stick when you try to carry a meal tray in a self-service restaurant, or jump quickly onto a tube train with crutches or sit in a confined aircraft seat with a rigid leg?

For the disabled, probably the most unkind feature of our towns and cities is the siting of public lavatories. Many are in basements or upstairs or in the most distant corner of clubs or restaurants. On trains it is often a feat of balance for even a fit person to enter the small cubicles. Where turnstiles exist it is impossible for a chairbound person to get to the lavatory without calling for special assistance from the attendant—who may not be present.

When a disabled person also has a urinary complication and must go frequently to the lavatory there is often no alternative but to stay at home.

Attitudes to the disabled

The general Public

Doctors, nurses and others who work in hospital among the disabled, and people who are similarly disabled, find such disability unremarkable and do not stare or comment when a person using crutches or a wheelchair passes by. Members of the public, unused to seeing disabled persons, wheelchairs, crutches often embarrass the disabled by giving unwanted assistance, staring, or avoiding the sight of the person. Much needs to be done to educate the public on the problems of the disabled. The disabled person is often happiest in an environment where there are many others with similar problems and where he is accepted as one of a crowd.

Nurses

Dame Agnes Hunt, who was pioneer in establishing welfare schemes for the disabled, defined 'Help, not pity', as the desirable attitude to the deformed or disabled. Pity is a useless attitude and most nurses do not demonstrate it. They should develop a positive approach that will help the person with a physical problem to improve his way of living and adjust to existence with a residual disability.

Employers

Most employers of labour will try to find work for a person with normal intellect provided the disability is moderate. Legislation exists that requires employers to use disabled employees if the factory or works is large enough, but this quota can be filled with blind persons or people with a mild degree of disability.

Taxation also militates against the employment of the physically handicapped. If taxation must be paid for every employee the manager of the works is obviously going to employ fit people who can work at a good rate of production.

Often the type of work, the location of the factory or the need for special concessions such as ground-floor employment, are problems, so that many disabled people devise their own form of employment at home. Watch repairing or electronic work are obvious examples. There are many voluntary societies who give help in the employment of the homebound disabled.

COMPENSATIONS

There are some physical compensations for being disabled. The patient who has lost the use of one or both legs often develops superb musculature around the shoulders and arms enabling him to use the arms to hoist himself from a chair or bed or to cover great distances on crutches.

Often, physically disabled folk will learn to use whatever is left in an unusual fashion. The use of the feet to write, draw, sew or dress is an example.

The patient's point of view

1.   How to live with a disability

This was written by a patient who has a completely rigid spine, including his neck. He does full time work with no concessions because he is disabled.

The title of this section is interesting because it immediately struck me that the dreadful alternative was 'Why let a disability kill you?' If this is the only alternative, a disabled person clearly has no choice—he must live with it. He should not be pitied on this score, but tactful, discreet help is always welcome.

The difficulties facing a severely disabled person need no amplification from me but one point omitted by the authors is the lack of reserve resources in the disabled person's physical ability. To give an example, the average person can climb a flight of stairs with little physical strain. The disabled person with lower limb disability can just get up with extreme effort. This is all well known but let the disabled person be unfortunate enough to get some trivial blister on his palm and his very mobility is immediately shattered because he can no longer use his crutches. This, to my mind, is one of the major frustrations of a disability—one gets by quite nicely, thank you, and then WHAM—a triviality becomes a disaster.

PSYCHOLOGY

To probe one's own outlook is dangerous—other classifications may be heaped on one's head—'introspective', 'neurotic', 'self-pitying'—but risking it for once I'll try to put myself on my own psychiatric couch and explain how I tick.

I think all disabled people have a chip on their shoulder about their disability and I do not like people to talk about my disability. I hate being asked 'What happened to you then?' I adore people who accept me as I am and do not fuss. I hate people who stare and even worse are those—usually on promenades at the seaside—who nudge their neighbours and one imagines the furtive whisper 'Just look at him' I'm afraid I'm rather rude about this as I usually stop and stare back though I'm never quite sure who is the more embarrassed they, I hope! The annoying thing about this particular aspect is that I know these very same people are basically kind and if I were to ask them for some help and it was within their power to help me they would do so willingly. Yet because I'm 'different' a wall of antipathy is thrown up by me against them.

WORK AND TRAVEL

I'm lucky—I have an interesting job in a wonderful organization. I feel that I do my duty as well as any 'normal' person in a similar capacity. This is supremely important as the things one does well one can enjoy and this means no frustration and the complete achievement of that feeling of independence so well described by the authors. Again I'm lucky where travelling is concerned. I can drive a car and take my family with me. My car is my Number 1 priority for material possessions. It is the door to the outside world and to me represents my job, my freedom of mobility and—here comes that chip again—it puts me on equal terms with the next bloke. We are all 'classified' by our contemporaries. Some are 'intellectual', 'mean', 'stupid', 'handsome', 'ugly', and so on *ad nauseam*. My category is 'disabled' but I get by quite well, thank you, What's yours?

2. Getting beneath the surface

This patient also has severe disability and is married to a registered nurse:

When I was asked to comment on this article I consented with some trepidation. Every persons is an individual and even disabilities of a similar nature can call for different application.

However, after putting up with a progressive condition for over twenty years and having experience of treatment in thirteen hospitals in this country I think I can give my own personal view with some justification. I agree with the basic principles of the chapter but feel the authors have, of necessity, only skimmed the surface.

PROBLEMS OF DEFORMITY

The problems of deformity can cover every form imaginable. If a time and motion study consultant was put on to me I think he would soon be asking for an appointment with a psychiatrist—for example, even the simple task of dressing, which takes a normal able-bodies person five minutes, requires one to one and a half hours of scheming with different aids and this does not include manoeuvring out of bed!

This will give you some idea of the time element involved, especially if you are keeping an appointment. Dressing can be made even more difficult by a drop in temperature in the depths of winter—with snow and ice outside the bedroom there can be much gnashing of teeth. Some efficient form of heating is therefore a great help.

Aids and appliances all have their uses and their limitations; they are only as useful as the disability will allow them to be. For example, with a hydraulic hoist the slings have to be put under the patient and nearly always operated by someone else. Wheelchairs may need pushing or even battery-driven ones need recharging, and with terminals low down underneath the chair this will create a problem. Add to this the fact that electric power points in most dwellings are at skirting-board level, and I think you will being to understand what I mean by limitations. There are innumerable examples I could quote, but to my mind they all have to be overcome. No doubt some day, with the help of medicine and technology, they will be overcome. Although most people think of appliances as technical problems I have purposely put medicine first, because by relieving the disability one can make more use of aids and appliances.

PAIN

Excruciating pain has to be contained within the confines of the mind. In my experience this can be achieved to a certain degree (a) by the help of the latest drug therapy, and (b) by intensive study or working to very fine limits at a subject which holds great interest. This latter can be even more important than the former, as the brain can be completely absorbed and the pain may be pushed into the background.

Nursing staff should realize that because a person does not complain, it does not mean that he is not in pain. Many disabled people give the impression of being in much less pain than they really are.

Health cannot be bought, but financial independence plays a major part in achieving independence in other ways.

I agree that a bungalow on the level is the best form of dwelling for most disabled people. The only thing I would add is a shower with thermostatic controls which I find much more convenient and less effort than struggling in and out of the bath even with the help of a hoist.

Some time ago the British Government issued a directive that all public buildings should be erected with suitable access points for the disabled. It is up to everyone concerned to ensure that this is carried out right from the planning stage.

I would like to endorse what the authors say about the employment of the disabled. Each firm of any size should take a number of handicapped persons wherever this is possible.

The disabled person should endeavour to associate with fit people as well as with his fellow disabled. Each group has a lot to learn from the other and mixing will help to break down any barriers which may exist.

Conclusions

Any disease, injury or disability can be conveniently considered in three phases or aspects: First, prevention, second, early treatment and third, treatment of the established condition. Although the latter two merge into each other there is need of different emphasis with priorities according to the the length of time the condition has been present.

For instance prevention of accidents leading to paralysis may be largely a matter of rules, regulations, training and discipline. Prevention of paralysis due to poliomyelitis is by prophylactic inoculation with dead virus (Salk) or attenuated virus (Sabin). Prevention of paralysis secondary to tuberculosis of the spine is achieved by improved public health measures, B.C.G., inoculation (Calmette-Guerin) and antibacterial antibiotics and chemotherapy.

The outstanding contributions to the prevention of paralysis have been made by laboratory workers and public health officials.

In contrast, the treatment of established paralysis has been promoted by clinicians and in this country the names of two outstanding pioneers dominate the scene, Sir Robert Jones and Professor Sir Ludwig Guttmann. Each possessed vision and the necessary personality to turn the vision into actuality, founding a tradition of patient care which has permanently affected our concepts of treatment. Each saw that even if you cannot cure paralysis you could restore the patient to independence, usefulness and happiness, i.e. by rehabilitation. To do this it was necessary to instil in the patient a desire to achieve these things, to make him see that much can be achieved even if he is never going to regain 'normality'.

Good nursing and medical care are essential to avoid complications such as deformities, contractures, bed sores and urinary infection. Splinting, physiotherapy, occupational therapy and other aids to independences also play an important part. Much of this book will be occupied with the treatment of established paralysis. This is not because we underestimate the importance of prevention and early treatment, but because these aspects or phases of the various conditions largely fall into the province of other disciplines. Later treatment is above all a question of team work and following in the footsteps of these two great pioneers— Robert Jones and Ludwig Guttmann.

2 : Basic Concepts in Paralysis: Relevant Anatomy and Physiology

The control of the body is carried out by the central nervous system which may be classified into two parts:

1 The central nervous system.
2 The peripheral nervous system (see Fig. 2.1).

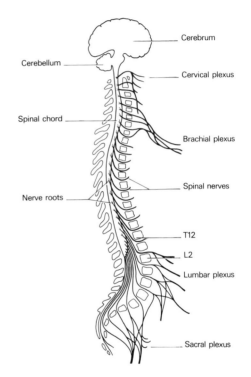

Cerebrum

Cerebellum

Cervical plexus

Spinal chord

Brachial plexus

Spinal nerves

Nerve roots

T12

L2

Lumbar plexus

Sacral plexus

Fig. 2.1. The central nervous system and peripheral nerves.

THE CENTRAL NERVOUS SYSTEM

The central nervous system is of outstanding importance in any animal body. It is very delicate and is the best-protected part. Indeed, any species which did not have a well-protected central nervous system would not survive in competition with others. In the human being, the covering is a hard bony case which totally encloses the vulnerable brain and spinal cord. The cranium, which encloses and protects the brain, is connected to the neural canal which surrounds the spinal cord. Inside the bony coverings are three membranes. The outer or dura mater, also known as the *theca*, (Fig. 2.2) extends around the brain and also from the skull to the lowest

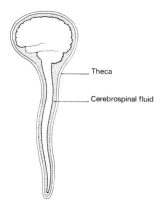

Fig. 2.2. The cavity containing the brain, spinal cord and cerebrospinal fluid; protected by the theca.

Theca

Cerebrospinal fluid

part of the vertebral column. Within the theca the brain and spinal cord are cushioned in fluid and membranes. The normal shocks of jumping, running or falling are not relayed to the central nervous system, but are dissipated over the fluid and membranes, i.e. the energy is diffused in both time and space so as to minimize the amount which reaches the nervous tissue. Even severe shocks are frequently accepted without causing damage to the brain and spinal cord. The internal volume of the theca is sufficient only for the contents. There is no reserve of space and the walls of the thecal space are inelastic.

Any substance which should not normally be there, such as a mass of clotted blood or a neoplasm, will occupy the volume which should be occupied by the nervous system. This is called a 'space-occupying' lesion. (Fig. 2.3). The effect is first to diminish the volume of blood in the thin-walled veins. If the lesion expands there will ultimately be cessation of the circulation, ischaemia, failure of function and ultimately death of the nerve cells which may lead to permanent paralysis, loss of the sensory and intellectual functions and the death of the patient.

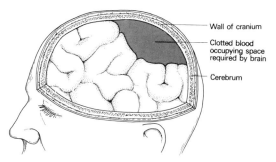

Wall of cranium

Clotted blood occupying space required by brain

Cerebrum

Fig. 2.3. A space-occupying lesion in the brain.

As the central nervous system is so carefully encased it is essential that there should be communicating pathways between the brain and spinal cord and the remainder of the body. These are the peripheral nerves. They are arranged into three groups:

1   Twelve pairs of cranial nerves.
2   Thirty-one pairs of spinal nerves.
3   A chain of sympathetic ganglia.

The cranial nerves are so called because they leave the upper cavity of the theca via openings in the cranial walls. They communicate between the organs such as the eyes, ears, nose and tongue and the central nervous system. (see Fig. 2.4).

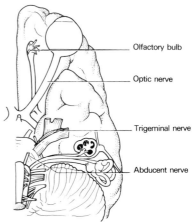

Olfactory bulb

Optic nerve

Trigeminal nerve

Abducent nerve

Fig. 2.4.   The cranial nerves leaving the cranium.

The spinal nerves are those which pass out of the vertebral column and communicate between the central nervous system and the muscles, skin, joints, bones, bowel, bladder and the other structures forming the human body. (see Fig. 2.5).

Additionally, *the sympathetic system* is a communicating network consisting of the sympathetic ganglia and sympathetic nerves which form a complex arrangement of nerve tissue around the exterior of the vertebral column. (see Fig. 2.6).

These communicating cranial and spinal nerves, consist of pathways which run towards the central nervous system (called 'afferent') and pathways going the other direction, away from the central nervous system (called 'efferent').

The afferent nerves transmit electrical impulses which convey data to the central nervous system about both external events and the internal events and working of the body. The efferent nerves carry impulses or messages from the central nervous system to all parts of the body. The

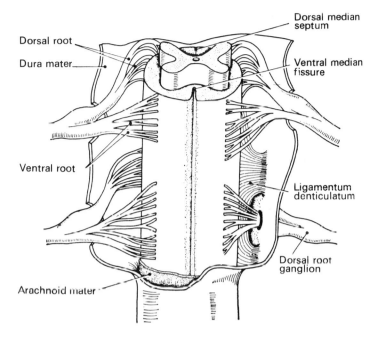

Dorsal median septum

Dorsal root

Dura mater

Ventral median fissure

Ventral root

Ligamentum denticulatum

Dorsal root ganglion

Arachnoid mater

Fig. 2.5.   Spinal nerves leaving the neural canal of the vertebral column, before passing to the muscles, skin, joints, bones, bowel, bladder, etc.

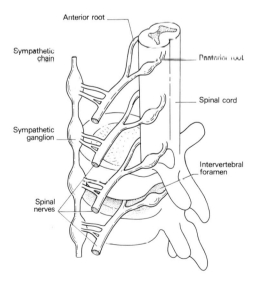

Anterior root

Sympathetic chain

Posterior root

Spinal cord

Sympathetic ganglion

Intervertebral foramen

Spinal nerves

Fig. 2.6.   The sympathetic ganglia on the vertebral column.

efferent impulses to the autonomic nervous system are carried out of the spinal canal by fibres closely associated with the motor nerves. It is necessary, in health, for all of these pathways to be complete and whole. Any interruption of the pathways results in severe disturbances of function of the central nervous system and therefore leads to severe problems for the patient. Any severance of the routes which connect the central nervous system to the rest of the body (the periphery) is called a 'peripheral nerve lesion', it may take any of several forms. (These are dealt with in Chapter 3.)

The peripheral nerves are bundles of nerve fibres. A nerve fibre projects from a nerve cell and is itself composed of protoplasm, similar to material composing the cell body (Fig. 2.7). The protoplasm is living material capable of the responses of such vital matter, respiration, assimilation of nutrition, reproduction and above all irritation. Thus, it responds to stimuli by transmitting them from one part of the nerve network to another. The bundles of nerve fibres, forming the peripheral nerves, are collected together into bundles by connective tissues. The connective tissue

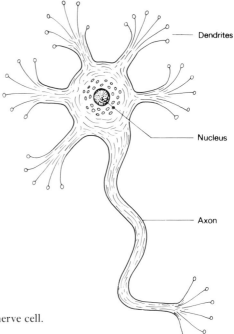

Fig. 2.7.   The structure of an efferent nerve cell.

serves as protection for the nerve and nerve fibres. Usually the protection is adequate to prevent damage to the nerves but when the trauma applied to the nerve is great, the protection is inadequate and the nerve is damaged. The degree of trauma is related to the amount of damage resulting. Thus a nerve may be bruised, crushed or completely severed. The distal fragment of the divided nerve fibre will disintegrate and ultimately disappear leaving an empty tube (each fibre is normally surrounded by what is known as a Schwann sheaths); this is known as Wallerian degeneration. This is discussed in more detail in Chapter 3.

The spinal cord

The spinal cord is a massive collection of nerve fibres collected into a trunk cables which are analogous to those used by the telephone engineer to connect one main exchange-junction to another. The spinal cord has many of the functions of a telephone system in that it transmits information of many kinds to the brain and returns instructions from the brain to the body. Thus within the spinal cord there are ascending pathways and descending pathways (Fig. 2.8). This description of the spinal cord tends to be too simple; it is truly a complex structure in which many activities besides transferring information occur. These will be discussed where they are relevant to conditions mentioned in other chapters.

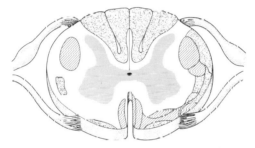

Fig. 2.8.   The ascending and descending pathways of the spinal cord. The ascending pathways are shaded. The descending pathways are stippled.

Although the spinal cord is well protected by bone and is surrounded by protective membranes and fluid it is still subject to damage by injury or disease. Again the effects of the damage will be related to the amount. Thus, the result may vary from minor problems of sensory or motor loss in the periphery of the body to a severe lesion with total loss of all function below the level of the transection.

The brain

The brain is at the upper end of the spinal cord and joins it at the junction of the cranium and the neural canal.

The part of the brain which connects the whole brain to the spinal cord is really a prolongation of the cord which is known as the medulla oblongata. It is of particular importance because it contains the vital centres responsible for breathing, coughing and sneezing; sucking, swallowing and vomiting; the rate and volume of the beat of the heart and the maintenance of blood pressure. Injury or disease affecting this part of the brain would result in malfunction or cessation of activities. The main mass of the brain is above the medulla oblongata. This is the largest portion of the central nervous system. It is mainly concerned with what are termed higher mental activities such as decision-making, taste, smell, memory, aesthetic sense and social awareness. The correct functioning of the cerebrum is closely connected with consciousness.

Muscles and posture

All active movement in the animal body is caused either directly or indirectly by muscle tissue. This ability, i.e. contractibility, makes muscle tissue shorten gently or forcefully. This reduction in length results in the application of force to the part or substance involved.

CARDIAC MUSCLE TISSUE

The heart walls move against the volume of blood inside its chambers. In contracting, the heart wall presses inwards on the contents of the heart at sufficient speed to squeeze the blood out and make the blood travel along the blood vessels with speed over a distance.

VISCERAL MUSCLE TISSUE

All the tubes of the body have the ability to alter the diameter of their lumen, because there is muscle tissue in the walls of the tubes which is arranged in two layers: one around the circumference and one along the length.

SKELETAL MUSCLE TISSUE

The bones and joints are moved by special tissue adapted to this function. The contractile tissue is arranged between two unstretchable attachments made of fibrous tissue, called tendons. There are many muscles firmly fixed to the periosteum (which surrounds bones) by specialized sheets of fibrous tissue called aponeuroses. When the contractile tissue pulls between two points, the relevant joint is moved (see Fig. 2.9).

Nerve and blood supply to muscle tissue

All classes of muscle tissue have some things in common. All need an excellent blood supply to function and are controlled by a nerve supply.

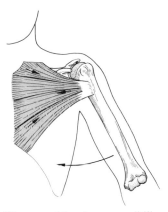

Fig. 2.9.   Muscle contractibility.

I   BLOOD SUPPLY

The blood supply to muscles is a major factor in their ability to function. In the process of working they require ample nutrition and oxygen (although when necessary they can function for a time without oxygen) and they must instantly excrete the wastes which would impede their function. (Impairment of blood supply is called ischaemia.)

2   NERVE SUPPLY TO MUSCLES

Control of muscle tissue is from the central nervous system (cardiac muscle can function independently when necessary) which exerts its influence via peripheral nerves. Impairment of the nerve supply to muscle tissue is called paralysis.

The neuromuscular junction

Skeletal muscles receive a nerve supply at a specialized area which is called the neuromuscular junction. At this point, the nerve supplying the muscle divides into a spray of branches which enter grooves in the muscle tissue. Stimulation from the nerve results in the release of a chemical called Acetylcholine. Acetylcholine has the function of causing the generalized contraction over all the fibres of the muscle.

There are diseases which are the result of lack of release of this chemical.

Deformities in paralysis

Deformity, that is, an unusual shape or position of part of the body, can

arise from a large number of causes. It may be due to intrinsic disorders
of the bone growth, failure of muscle growth or the effects of pathological
processes such as injuries, infections, tumours or destruction of tissue. A
very common cause of deformity is paralysis, i.e. any condition in which
the normal balance between muscles controlling the positions of the joints,
is upset. Unequal muscle action may cause deformities in many parts of the
body. For instance, unequal muscle action may cause a deformity of the
neck called torticollis, and this in turn, may be due to contracture of the
muscle as in so-called sternomastoid torticollis which used to be a common
condition in infancy, or it may be due to spasmodic contractions of the
muscle as in a large variety of diseases of the central nervous system, including athetosis, Parkinsonism, and that ill-understood condition, spasmodic
torticollis.

Chronic repeated contractions of muscles can in turn, lead to contracture,
i.e. permanent shortening of the muscles and to fibrosis and ultimately,
fibrotic changes in the joint capsule and limitation of movement. Abnormal
muscle contractions occurring in infancy can lead to disorders of growth
and even to premature fusion of the epiphyses and ankylosis of the joints.
Similarly, in other parts of the trunk, unequal action of muscles, due to
disorders of the central nervous system, the peripheral nerves of the
muscles or connective tissues, may lead to severe deformities such as
kyphosis, lordosis or scoliosis. It is particularly in the hands and feet that
neuromuscular disorders lead to severe deformities. These are worthy of a
special heading of their own.

Hand deformities due to muscle paralysis

As in other parts of the body, hand deformities may be due to a variety
of bone diseases, for example, tumours, osteomyelitis or tuberculosis.
There may be widespread destruction of joints as in rheumatoid arthritis,
or contracture of skin and fascia as in conditions like Duputyren's contracture. Contracture may occur as a secondary effect of burns or infection.
Various types of muscle paralysis classically produce well-hand deformities.

CLAW HAND

Muscle paralysis causes the doformity known as ulnar claw hand, in
which there is hyperextension of the metacarpo-phalangeal joints. particularly of the ring and little fingers. There is also hyperflexion of fixed deformity of the interphalangeal joints of the same fingers. This condition is
basically due to paralysis or weakness of the intrinsic muscles of the hand,

namely, the lumbricals and the interosseous muscles. Their primary function of these muscles is the flexion of the metacarpo-phalangeal joints and extension of the interphalangeal joints. Therefore, if they are weak or paralysed the unopposed long extensor tendons produce extension of the metacarpo-phalangeal joints and the unopposed long flexor tendons produce flexion of the interphalangeal joints. Not every patient with weakness of the intrinsic muscles develops this deformity, but it is especially likely to develop in children or women with very mobile hands. To a certain extent, it can be prevented by keeping the metacarpo-phalangeal joints slightly flexed. Under these circumstances, the long extensor tendons have some action on the interphalangeal joint and will extend them against the opposing action of the long flexor tendons. Both physiotherapy and splinting may, therefore, be employed to prevent a claw hand developing, even in the presence of ulnar paralysis.

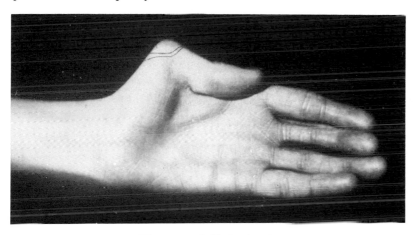

Fig. 2.10.   A Simian hand.

SIMIAN HAND

The next common deformity is the so-called Simian hand which is due to paralysis of the median nerve. The small muscles of the thumb are then weak or paralysed and the patient is no longer able to oppose and abduct the thumb. The thumb falls back into the same plane as the palm producing the flat or Simian hand. If the median nerve is damaged at a higher level, that is, if the long flexor tendons and muscles to the thumb and index finger are also involved, the patient will be unable to flex these and they will be held in the straight or pointing position. A combination of median and ulnar paralysis will produce a very flat Simian hand with clawing of all digits and dropping back of the thumb.

WRIST DROP

If the radial nerve is involved, there will be paralysis of the extensor muscles of the wrist, fingers and thumb, producing a so-called wrist drop, which may ultimately result in a permanent flexion deformity of both the fingers and wrist. If the posterior interosseous nerve alone is involved, then there will be paralysis of the finger and thumb extensors, but not of the radial wrist extensors, in which case the wrist will be held in dorsi-flexion and radial deviation, but the fingers will be flexed at the metacarpo-phalangeal joint.

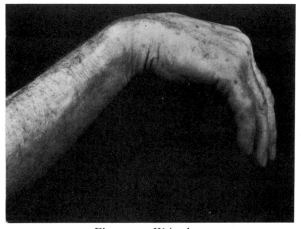

Fig. 2.11. Wrist drop.

SPASTIC HAND

In the presence of a spastic paralysis, the wrist and fingers are often held flexed. In extreme cases, the thumb will be flexed and adducted across the palm of the hand. Therefore, in the normal action of gripping, instead of the fingers coming in contact with the palm, the thumb will be interposed between the fingers and the thumb preventing normal gripping action. Occasionally, the fingers become so flexed that the finger tips press into the palm of the hand producing sores. There may be great difficulty in cleaning and washing the hand, and elementary toilet such as cutting the nails. In addition, in spastic conditions, it is uncommon for the forearm to be held in a fully pronated position and the elbow to be held flexed.

Foot deformities

The commonest foot deformity is the equinus deformity. This may be due either to overaction of the calf muscles as is seen in many types of

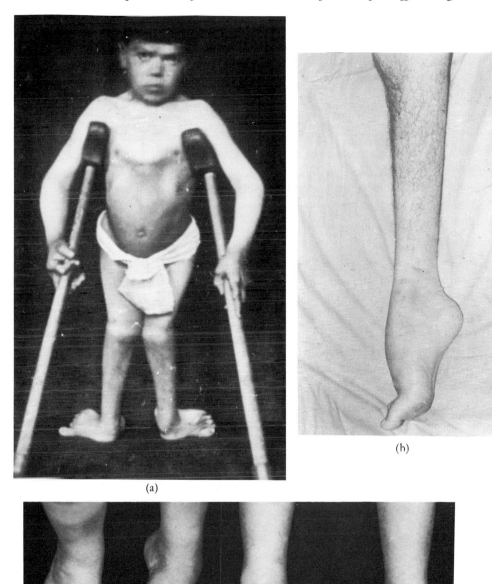

(a)

(h)

(c)

Fig. 2.12. *a:* Valgus or everted foot. *b:* Equinus foot. *c:* Inverted foot. Congenital talipes equino-varus. Superior and posterior aspects.

spastic paralysis or upper motor neurone lesions, or it may be due to weakness of the dorsiflexor muscles as is seen often in poliomyelitis and in lesions of the external popliteal nerve. Associated with an equinus deformity or foot drop, there is often inversion of the foot, often called a varus deformity. The foot assumes a position of equino-varus. This is because one of the important muscles, the tibialis posterior, is supplied by the posterior tibial nerve and is often not involved, even though the dorsiflexor and everter or anterior muscles are weak or paralysed. In addition, once the foot becomes inverted, the calf muscles acting through the tendo achilles, assume an inverting action thus increasing the deformity. The opposite deformity of a severely valgus or everted foot (Fig. 2.12a) is seen when there is weakness or paralysis of the invertor muscles, that is, the tibialis anterior and the tibialis posterior. In all foot deformities, once the deformity is present the delicate muscle balance is upset and the deformity is often progressive.

Another deformity which used to be commonly seen is the so-called calcaneous foot (Fig. 2.14), that is, excessive dorsiflexion which results from

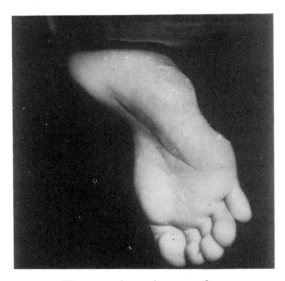

Fig.2.13.   An equino-cavus foot.

paralysis of the calf muscle. (Fig. 2.16). A similar deformity can be seen if there has been overlengthening of the tendo achilles, for instance, after surgical treatment of spastic paralysis. The deformity can also be produced by external forces applied to the foot of the growing child, as was classically seen in the feet of high-class Chinese girls, which had been bound since birth. Associated with the so-called calcaneous deformity, there may also be a cavus deformity, a condition in which the normal arch of the foot is increased or the forefoot is dropped in relation to the hindfoot, and the combination of the two is known as a calcaneo-cavus foot (Fig. 2.14). Cavus deformity of the foot is usually associated with hammer toes or clawing of the toes, i.e. hyperextension at the metatarso-phalangeal joints and flexion of the interphalangeal joints. This deformity occurs in a large number of neurological conditions such as spina bifida, seringo myelia, peroneal muscular atrophy, Friedrich's ataxia and so on. There has been considerable controversy about the nature and causation of the deformity.

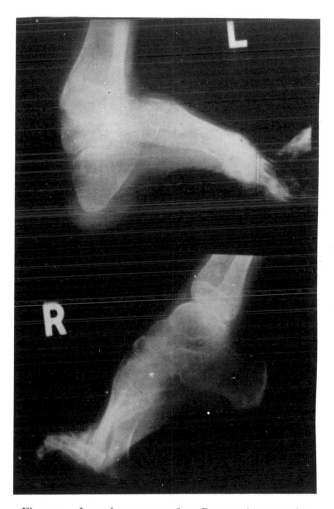

Fig. 2.14.   L, a calcaneo-cavus foot; R, an equino-cavus foot.

It is known that the toes are normally balanced rather precariously on the heads of the metatarsal, and as in the hands, the interosseous and lumbrical muscles act as planter flexors at the metacarpo-phalangeal joints and extensors of the interphalangeal joints. The long flexor muscles act as flexors of the interphalangeal joints and the so-called extensors of the toes act as extensors at the metatarso-phalangeal joints. If anything upsets this delicate balance, the toes become deformed. Once there has been hyperextension at the metatarso-phalangeal joints or even a subluxation, the intrinsic muscles become displaced dorsally and take on an altered function. Instead of acting as flexors of the metatarso-phalangeal joints, they act as extensors and a vicious circle is established which leads to increase of the deformity. There are, of course, other muscles involved. For instance, the peroneal muscles, tibilias anterior and the tibialis posterior are all responsible for holding up the arch of the foot. If their action becomes unbalanced they can lead to raising of the arch or pes cavus. When the metatarsal heads become dropped, the extensor muscles of the front of the leg which contribute to dorsiflexion of the foot now acting on the already subluxated proximal phalanges, increase the displacement of the toes instead of lifting the whole of the forefoot. The result is that the metatarsal heads drop still further and the proximal phalanges become still further displaced dorsally.

Knee deformities

The commonest deformity of the knee is a flexion deformity, due either to paralysis of the quadriceps muscle or to overaction of the hamstring muscles as is seen in a large variety of types of spastic paralysis. Occasionally, the opposite deformity of hyperextension or limitation of flexion of the knee is seen. This can occur either because there is an active quadriceps muscle with paralysed ham string muscles, or it can be due to fibrosis in the quadriceps muscle. This fibrosis may be a result of a constitutional condition like arthrogryposis, or it may be secondary to injection of antibiotics into the thigh during infancy. It may be a congenital deformity. Equinus deformity of the foot aggravates genu recurvatum.

Hip deformities

The commonest deformity in the hip, is a flexion and adduction deformity, due to relative increase in strength of the flexor and adductor muscles, as in spastic paralysis or a lower motor neurone paralysis of the gluteal muscles. This deformity is especially sinister because it may lead

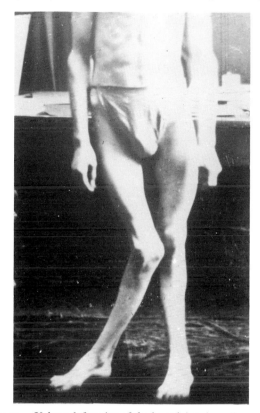

Fig. 2.15. Valgus deformity of the knee joints in poliomyelitis.

to dislocation of the hip with very dire consequences, the leg becoming shorter and weaker, the hip becoming painful and the leg being permanently flexed and adducted.

THE GENERAL CARE OF THE PARALYSED PATIENT

Patients with severe paralysis require specialized management which can only be supplied by a team of individuals working together. There are many aspects of care which can only be offered in special units in hospitals which inadequate neurological, spinal injury, cerebral palsy or orthopaedic centres.

The team

The work of the supervising doctor must be supported by many ancillary services. Paralysed patients require prolonged treatment and follow-up.

An infant born with a neurological disorder must commence treatment soon after birth and the care must then continue until the child is an adult. This form of treatment can only be maintained in a community when it is served by a team of doctors, nurses, radiographers, occupational therapists, social caseworkers, pharmacists, pathology technicians, stenographers, clerical records staff and many others who, though they may not be directly involved in the treatment of the patient, are essential for efficient care.

AFTERCARE AND COMMUNITY FOLLOW-UP CARE

All the dedicated work of the hospital team is futile unless some form of care is given when the patient has left hospital and is in his home, which may be a great distance from the central hospital. The care may be the continuation of the specialized management of the particular unit by a team that travels to the home of the patient, or holds clinics in premises adjacent to the place where the patient lives. The most likely and consistent daily care will probably be given by the general practitioner responsible for the general welfare of the patient supported by visiting community nurses, physiotherapists and occupational therapists. It is essential in the latter circumstances to ensure that there is full communication between the hospital and the community services. Full communication between all members of the hospital team and their counterparts in the community must occur before the patient is due for discharge from the hospital and continuously after return to his home environment and possibly to employment.

Physiotherapy in paralysis

The aim of physiotherapy in paralysis is threefold: first of all to prevent deformity; secondly, to preserve joint mobility; and thirdly, to aid the restoration of normal muscle function.

The prevention of deformity in the presence of paralysis may be achieved by active exercises, assisted exercises, passive movements or splinting. There is a role for each of these. In the presence of total flaccid paralysis, joint mobility and the prevention of deformity can only be achieved by passive movements. In the presence of spasticity, passive movements have to be performed with great gentleness, otherwise they may, by initiating stretch reflexes, increase the spasm. The highly skilled physiotherapist has the ability to help the patient put his or her joints through a full range of movements without initiating harmful spasm. Indeed, the skilled physiotherapist can often manipulate the joints so that beneficial reflex actions result rather than harmful ones. In a simple flaccid paralysis, splinting can be used to prevent deformity but of course, it must be used with discretion, as otherwise it may lead to stiffness of joints or prevent the patient from trying to use the limb within the limits of his or her muscle power. In the presence of spasticity, splinting is a very double-edged weapon as it may initiate painful reflex spasms leading to the development of pressure sores and worse trouble. Therefore, the use of any type of splinting in spastic or upper motor neurone paralysis has to be approached with great care, caution and insight. There is, however, considerable evidence that correct positioning of limbs, especially in the early stages, helps to determine the pattern of reflex action in the future. If the position of the limbs is neglected, for instance, in traumatic paraplegia, then not only do the limbs become contracted, but the patient is much more likely to develop painful flexor spasms. With correct positioning, deformities will not develop and the likelihood of troublesome flexor or adductor spasms developing is very much less. We do not understand all the factors which lead to the development of flexor spasms but they are basically due to certain unopposed spinal reflexes. These reflexes are normally inhibited by the integrity of the long tract in the spinal cord leading from the brain to the anterior horn cells. We do know that a number of extrinsic factors such as poor health, infection, distension of the bladder or bowel, pressure sores, emotional disturbances and so on, seem to have a deleterious effect and increase the tendency towards harmful flexor spasms. A great deal of the success of a skilled physiotherapist will lie in inhibiting the flexor spasm and the developing of beneficial reflex responses. The restoration of muscle activity after paralysis entirely rests on factors outside the physiotherapist's control, for instance if there has been damage to a peripheral nerve, ultimate restoration of muscle function depends on new axon fibres growing down to the motor endplate of the muscle. During the waiting period when it is hoped that nerve function will be restored, there is some evidence that galvanic stimulation of the muscles will prevent them atrophying, and improve the chances of useful function being restored. Unfortunately, for such treatment to be effective it must be conducted daily and for at least an hour a day. This of course, is not practical in most cases, though for selected patients they can be lent their own equipment.

General principles in the nursing of paralysed parts

The nursing care required by the paralysed patient depends upon the degree of the paralysis. The patient with tetraplegia, hemiplegia or paraplegia (see Chapter 5) requires intensive nursing in the first stages. Less intensive nursing is required as the patient progresses towards rehabilitation and independence. The person with a peripheral nerve lesion (see Chapter 3) causing monoplegia or weakness of a muscle or group of muscles will also require less intensive care. Certain basic principles concerning the nursing care of the parts which are paralysed must be stated and followed in all cases, :–

1　VULNERABILITY

As the patient's central nervous system does not receive afferent impulses from the skin of the paralysed part no reflex or voluntary action is made which would protect it from damage. Indeed, the patient may not be able to take any form of action to protect the paralysed part.

2　TEMPERATURE CONTROL

In health, the volume of blood in a limb increases or decreases in response to need. If a part increases or decreases in temperature because of radiation or contact from warmer surroundings there is an instant physiological response to adjust the temperature to that of the rest of the body. Because of paralysis, this vasomotor control of the blood in the limb is lost and the area is more susceptible to heat or coldness.

It is therefore necessary to protect the part from these extremes. The paralysed hand of a patient should be gloved and the arm protected by a sleeve in cold weather even though the patient does not complain of the cold, if frostbite is to be avoided. It is unwise for the patient to sit or lie near a source of heat such as an electric bar fire, electric blanket or hot water bottle. A more diffuse form of heating is safer.

3　FRICTION SORES

Because the part is anaesthetic, the tissues flaccid and without tone and resistance to pressure, the tissues are more susceptible to injury from minor trauma. The rough edge of a sleeve rubbing against the wrist, or the crease in a sock or the stone inside the shoe can result in sores which require extended treatment for healing to occur. Therefore, constant awareness of these possibilities is essential both by the attendants and the patient.

4　PRESSURE ULCERATION

Constant pressure on the paralysed area must be avoided, as stated above. The seated patient is taught 'press-ups' (see Fig. 5.16) and care must always be taken to ensure that a paralysed limb is not overlain by the leg.

5   GRAVITATIONAL PROBLEMS

Because vasomotor responses do not occur in the paralysed part in re-action to an alteration in position there is a tendency for blood to rush into a paralysed part in response to gravity. Thus one area of the body will be engorged with blood whilst another is deprived of blood. This deprived area may be the brain. It is unwise to permit a paralysed limb to hang dependently (for example an arm hanging over the side of a bed or couch). It is essential to be aware that some tetraplegic patients cannot tolerate sudden alteration in posture or do not enjoy being seated upright for too long.

The good nursing management of a paralysed appendage requires:

1   Constant observation to note changes in the skin colour, skin tempera-ture or shape of the part.

2   Careful protection of the limb from heat, cold or injury.

3   Support for the limb to avoid gravitational engorgement when the limb is dependent.

4   Careful placing when the patient is recumbent to avoid compression from another part of the body.

5   Full toiletry of the whole limb with careful washing and drying each day, particularly where two skin surfaces are in contact, dusting lightly with talc and manicure by someone other than the patient.

6   Physiotherapy to carry out passive movements of all affected joints and to note any return of function.

7   Removal of splintage for cleaning and regular maintenance. Replace-ment must be considered when necessary.

3 : Peripheral Nerve Lesions

Definition

A peripheral nerve is a nerve trunk which communicates between the central nervous system (the brain and spinal cord inside the theca) and the periphery of the body (the parts outside the theca, e.g. muscles, and skin) (Fig. 3.1). The cranial and spinal nerves which together comprise the peripheral nerves, are the routes by which nervous impulses arising in the brain and spinal cord pass in and out to supply the skin, muscles, bones, blood vessels, glands, sensory organs and other structures of the body. Damage to these nerves therefore results in an interruption in the communicating pathway connecting the brain and spinal cord with the periphery of the body. Such an interruption is called a peripheral nerve lesion.

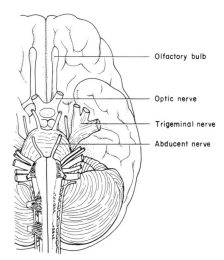

Olfactory bulb

Optic nerve

Trigeminal nerve

Abducent nerve

Fig. 3.1. The cranial nerves leaving the cranium.

Each peripheral nerve consists of three types of fibres:
1 Motor or afferent fibres—i.e. the fibres which conduct nervous impulses from the spinal cord to the striated muscles.
2 Sensory or afferent fibres—which conduct nervous impulses from peripheral sense organs, e.g. sensory receptors in the skin, muscles, joints and tendons to the spinal cord.
3 Autonomic fibres which conduct impulses from the spinal cord to the sweat glands, blood vessels and hairs.

32

Lesions of peripheral nerves can interfere with one or all of these functions either completely or partly. Complete division of a peripheral nerve produces firstly, paralysis and ultimately, wasting of the muscles supplied by that nerve; secondly, loss of sensation in the area of skin normally supplied by the nerve, and thirdly, absence of sweating and impairment of vasomotor control in the same distribution as the area of sensory loss.

The nerves which are classified as peripheral nerves are the twelve pairs of cranial nerves and the thirty-one pairs of spinal nerves (Fig. 3.2.).

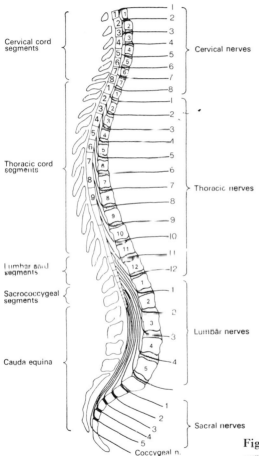

Fig. 3.2. Thirty-one pairs of spinal nerves leaving the vertebral column.

The cranial nerves

There are twelve pairs of nerves which pass out of the cranial cavity to the periphery. In this case the periphery is mainly the area adjacent to the skull. Thus these nerves connect the brain with (1) the important organs of sight, smell, taste and hearing, (2) the muscles of facial expression, eye control and head position and (3) the viscera through the vagus nerve. Most of them therefore have only a short distance to cover but must pass through openings in the bony cranium to reach or return from their objective. Thus they are vulnerable in injuries affecting the face, head and neck. A common event in severe fractures of the facial or cranial bones is loss of one of the functions to which the cranial nerves contribute. They are, of course, also subject to impairment of function due to infections, chemical toxins and new growths. Some pharmacological preparations used in therapy have side effects which may cause cranial nerve irritation or palsy.

The cranial nerves are classified as shown in Table 3.1.

Table 3.1.   Classification of the cranial nerves.

Number	Name of cranial nerve	Function of the nerve	Results of a lesion affecting the nerve
I	Olfactory nerve	*Sensory* from the nasal cavities.	Impairment or loss of the sense of smell. This is associated with reduced sense of taste.
2	Optic nerve	*Sensory* from the retina of the eye. The nerve of sight.	Impairment or loss of vision.
3	Oculomotor nerve	*Motor* to: (a) the muscles which move the eye. (b) the muscles inside the eye which alter the size of the pupil.	Convergent, divergent or concommitant strabismus (squint). Loss of control of the amount of light reaching the retina.
4	Trochlear nerve	*Motor* to one of the muscles which move the eye.	
5	Trigeminal nerve Ophthalmic branch (forms three sub-branches).	*Sensory* from: (a) Cornea of the eye (b) Ciliary body of the eye (c) Iris of the eye (d) Lacrimal gland (e) Conjuntiva of the eye (f) Nasal cavity. (g) Skin of eyelid, eyebrow, forehead and nose.	Anaesthesia affecting the parts listed.

Table 3.1. (contd.)

Number	Name of cranial nerve	Function of the nerve	Results of a lesion affecting the nerve
5	Trigeminal nerve Maxillary branch	*Sensory* from: (a) Dura mater inside cranial cavity. (b) The forehead. (c) Lower eyelid. (d) Lateral angle of the orbital cavity. (e) The upper lip. (f) The gums and teeth of the upper jaw. (g) The mucous membrane and skin of the cheek and nose.	Anaesthesia of the parts listed.
5	Trigeminal nerve (c) Mandibular branch.	*Sensory* from: (a) The temple. (b) The pinna of the ear. (c) The lower lip. (d) Lower part of the face. (e) Teeth and gums of the mandible. (f) Mucous membrane of the anterior of the tongue (taste)	Anaesthesia of the parts listed.
		Motor to: The muscles of mastication.	Weakness or paralysis of the muscles controlling the mandible results in loss of ability to close jaw and bite.
6	The abducent nerve.	*Motor* to one of the muscles which move the eye.	Weakness of lateral movements of the eyelid.
7	The facial nerve.	*Sensory* from: (a) The anterior two-thirds of the tongue (taste). (b) Middle ear. *Motor* to: (a) Sublingual glands. (b) Submaxillary glands.	Loss of some taste. Anaesthesia of the parts named.

Table 3.1. (contd.)

Number	Name of cranial nerve	Function of the nerve	Results of a lesion affecting the nerve.
		(c) Muscles of the face. (d) Part of the scalp. (e) The pinna of the ear. (f) The muscles of the neck.	Facial paralysis.
8	The acoustic (auditory) nerve.	*Sensory* with two functions: (a) *The cochlear branch* is the nerve of hearing.	Reduction or loss of hearing in the affected ear.
		(b) *The vestibular branch* is the nerve of balance.	Problems related to equilibrium, such as dizziness (vertigo) or difficulties related to positioning of the head in space.
9	The vagus nerve.	The cranial nerve with the widest distribution of branches throughout the neck, thorax and abdomen. *Motor fibres* to: (a) The muscles of the pharynx. (b) The muscles of the larynx. (c) The muscles of the trachea. (d) The heart. (e) The larger arteries and veins. (f) The arch of the aorta.	Problems related to interference with the autonomic nervous system.
		(g) The oesophagus. (h) The stomach. (i) The small intestine. (j) Pancreas. (k) The liver. (l) The spleen. (m) The ascending colon. (n) Kidneys (o) Visceral blood vessels.	

Table 3.1. (contd.)

Number	Name of cranial nerve	Function of the nerve	Results of a lesion affecting the nerve.
10	Vagus nerve.	*Sensory fibres* from: (a) Mucous membrane of the larynx. (b) Mucous membrane the trachea. (c) The lungs. (d) The oesophagus. (e) The stomach. (f) The intestines. (g) The gall bladder.	Problems related to disturbance of the autonomic nervous system.
11	The accessory nerve	*Motor* with two parts: (a) *Cranial* to the pharynx and larynx. (b) *Spinal* to the sterno-cleido-mastoid muscle and trapezius muscle.	Disturbance of the autonomic nervous system. Paralysis of these muscles.
12	The hypoglossal nerve.	*Motor* to the muscles of the tonge and the lyoid bone.	Paralysis affecting the tongue

The spinal nerves

The spinal nerves arise at different segmental levels of the spinal cord (Fig. 3.3). There are eight cervical, twelve dorsal, five lumbar, five sacral and one coccygeal pair. As the cord terminates at the highest part of the lumbar region, the nerves leaving the lower part of the spinal cord must pass down inside the spinal canal before they pass through the spinal foramina and thence to the peripheral organs.

Each of the spinal nerves arise from the cord by two nerve roots on each side of the cord. The root at the front transmits the impulses going out to the body (efferent or motor root), the root at the back transfers the impulses received from the body into the cord and brain (afferent or sensory root). Normally these roots are related to a pathway going up the cord to the brain (the posterior sensory root) or a pathway coming down the cord from the brain (the anterior motor root). Communication between the posterior root and the anterior root by communicating neurones within the spinal

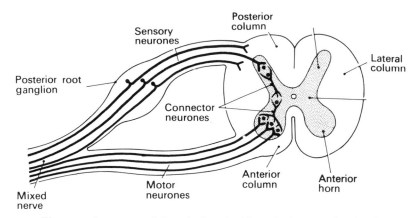

Fig. 3.3. A segment of the spinal cord with a spinal nerve related to it.

cord also occurs. The functional combination of sensory organ afferent nerve, communicating neurone or neurones, afferent nerve and the muscle it supplies is known as a reflex arc. (Fig. 3.4.) An automatic motor response elicited by stimulating a sensory end organ and utilizing a reflex arc is known as a reflex action.

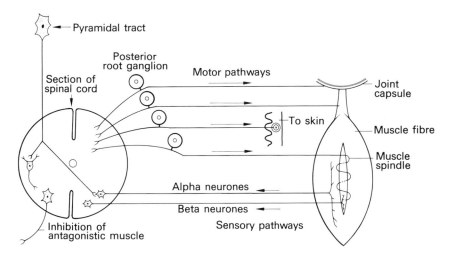

Fig. 3.4. The reflex arcs, which control movement.

THE PLEXUSES

The spinal nerves are grouped together at certain levels particularly where they serve a limb. This grouping is the basis for the formation of many branches which supply a number of different structures arising from a few nerve roots. The main plexuses are:

1 The cervical plexus. This supplies the muscles and structures of the neck. (Fig. 3.5).

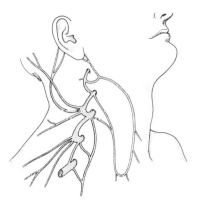

Fig. 3.5. The cervical plexus related to the neck.

2   The brachial plexus. This supplies the upper extremity including the muscles connecting the thorax and the scapula, the shoulder, the arm and the hand. The plexus is situated in the antero lateral part of the neck and superior and medial to the shoulder joint, i.e. just above and behind the clavicle. It may be damaged by wounds or injuries in this area. (Fig. 3 6).

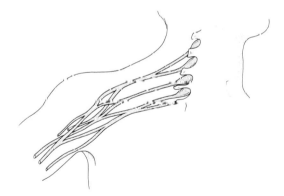

Fig. 3.6. The brachial plexus related to the neck and shoulder.

3   The lumbar plexus. (Fig. 3.7). This is situated at the back of the abdominal cavity on the side of the vertebral column. It passes forwards to supply the anterior, lateral and medial surface of the thigh and the anterior muscles of the hip and thigh. It may be damaged by wounds of the abdominical cavity or back.

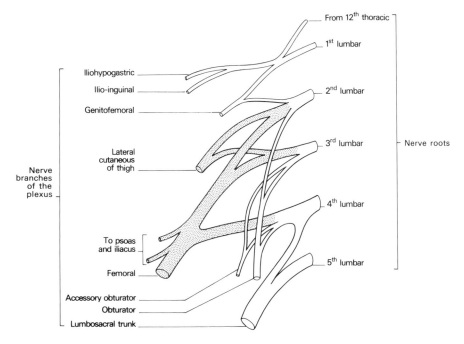

Fig. 3.7. The lumbar plexus.

4   The sacral plexus. This is situated within the pelvis on the anterior surface of the sacrum. The largest branch passes out through the great sciatic notch at the back of the pelvis. It may be damaged in fractures and other injuries of the pelvis. The sacral plexus supplies the skin at the back of the thigh and the skin of the leg and foot below the knee. It supplies all the muscles below the knee and the back of the thigh and buttock. (Fig. 3.8).

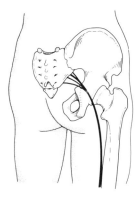

Fig. 3.8.   The sacral plexus related to the buttock.

Lesions affecting the plexuses

The grouping of nerve roots to form nerve branches results in the formation of a mass of nerve tissue in particular areas of the neck and trunk. There is such a mass at the base of the neck, at the side of the lumbar region of the vertebral column and on the antero-lateral surface of the sacrum in the pelvis. As these parts are vulnerable to trauma in gunshot wounds, industrial and transportation accidents the relevant plexus is often also included in the lesion. This can result in severance, avulsion, or crushing of any part of the plexus with consequent paralysis of the limb or part of the limb served by the plexus. Thus an injury in the region of the neck can cause paralysis and anaesthesia in the arm and hand and an injury in the abdominal or pelvic region can result in weakness or paralysis of the relevant leg or foot.

The importance of peripheral nerve lesions

Lesions of peripheral nerves are mainly of economic and personal importance. By themselves, they do not usually lead directly to loss of life or permanent ill-health, although indirectly they may if complications such as infection supervene. However, they interfere very considerably with an individual's functional attainments, that is, his ability to look after himself and his personal needs, to take part in sport and recreations and to earn a living. Naturally, the relative importance varies according to the patient's age, sex, occupation and interests and the nerve involved. Lesions of peripheral nerves, may arise from a vast number of different causes. In times of war, gunshot wounds are very common causes. In certain countries stab wounds due to riots or criminal assaults, are increasingly common. Among children, falls and cuts are common causes of peripheral nerve lesions. The increased mechanization both of transport and industrial processes has also led to a vast increase in peripheral nerve lesions. In certain industries, which use a large number of machines with sharp cutting edges or rotating tools, lesions of the peripheral nerve often occur. In victims of motor accidents, (occupants of cars or pedestrians) peripheral nerve lesions are not uncommon. In many fracture dislocations, damage to a peripheral nerve is an important associated injury. Indeed, one might say that in any given fracture or dislocation it is not so much the fracture or the dislocation itself which is likely to lead to serious permanent disability, but associated lesions which damage the peripheral nerves.

As mentioned earlier, the peripheral nerve lesions seldom give rise to loss of life or even by themselves, to loss of limb, but of course, peripheral

nerve lesions may be associated with damage to blood vessels or skin and
this may lead ultimately to loss of a limb due to ischaemia. Also, if there is
widespread impairment of sensation this may lead to formation of ulcers
which become infected and ultimately chronic infection and osteomyelitis
may impair health and necessitate amputation.

The classification of peripheral nerve lesions (Fig. 3.9)

An ideal classification should be comprehensive, consistent and constructive. Comprehensiveness means that all the possible pathological
conditions are included. Consistency means that the classification is based
on comparable and related criteria, for instance, a classification might be
based on regional anatomy, or on the aetiological agent concerned. Sometimes one bases a classification on the circumstances of the injury, for
instance, a certain type of radial nerve paralysis which was attributed to a
patient falling asleep with his arm over the back of a chair in a drunken
stupor, was known as Saturday night paralysis. It would, in a sense, be
perfectly consistent to classify all injuries by the day of the week and the
time of the day at which they occurred, but of course, this would not
necessarily be very constructive, meaning the classification should be
helpful in arriving at a full pathological diagnosis and prognosis which of
course, are the basies on which all treatment must be based. Any given

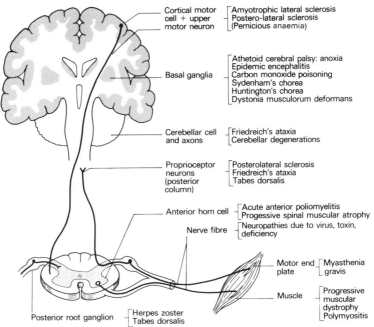

Fig. 3.9.   Diseases of specific structures of the nervous system.

peripheral nerve consists of a collection of nerve fibres. There are motor fibres of varying diameters, sensory fibres with different diameters and functions, and there are autonomic fibres. Any given nerve fibre may be in one of four conditions. (1) It may be intact and conducting normally. (2) It may be anatomically intact but temporarily not functioning, that is, there is a physiological block to conduction. (3) There may be an interruption of the axon sheath but the nerve sheath is intact, i.e. the axon distal to the site of the lesion will undergo Wallerian degeneration (see page 47) but eventually the proximal part of the axon, (that is the part in contact with the nerve cell) will grow down the nerve sheaths replacing the degenerating peripheral part. Ultimately, there will be restoration of function without the necessity for surgical intervention (Fig. 3.10). Lastly, (4) both nerve sheath and the axon fibre may be divided, under which circumstances unless the two severed ends of the nerve fibre are brought into contact, there will be no regeneration and recovery. Perhaps one should add a fifth state of the nerve, namely one in which the nerve is being irritated. This however, is to a large extent a clinical concept rather than a pathological concept because the nerve is in a sense functioning normally, conducting impulses, but either due to external stimulus or to a breakdown of internal insulation, stimuli and impulses are irritating the nerve causing either pain or spontaneous muscle action and fasciculation. This clinical syndrome may be mimicked by lesions of the central nervous system. The aim of the clinician is, to diagnose the exact condition of each nerve fibre. This ideal is, however, seldom attainable. Therefore, although we are aiming at what might be termed a micropathological diagnosis which indicates the exact condition of every nerve fibre in a given nerve, in the early stages by clinical examination alone, we can only make a provisional diagnosis. Perhaps the simplest and most important provisional diagnosis to make is to decide whether the majority of the nerve fibres in the peripheral nerve have intact neuro-

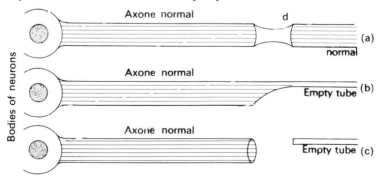

Fig. 3.10.   Types of nerve lesions. (a) Axonotmesis with continuity; neurotmesis (b) with apparent continuity due to stretching and (c) with no continuity.

sheaths, that is if spontaneous recovery is likely to occur, or whether the majority or a significant number if the nerve fibres have been completely divided. If there is a separation of the nerve ends the probability is that the loss of the function will be permanent unless some measures are taken to bring the severed nerve ends into approximation. There are a number of factors which must be taken into account in trying to make this provisional diagnosis. Clearly, one of these is the type of injury; a nerve lesion where there is complete loss of motor, sensory and autonomic function is more likely to be irrecoverable if it is associated with an open wound such as a cut or gunshot wound. If it is associated with a closed fracture, or if the injury is due to a traction force or to the injection of a noxious chemical compound into the nerve, it is less likely to lead to permanent paralysis and loss of function. So, one has to decide whether the lesion is physiologically complete because a complete lesion is much more likely to represent complete division of the nerve than an incomplete lesion and then consider the mechanism of the injury to make a good guess about the exact state of the nerve. Of course, immediately after an injury to a peripheral nerve there may be complete loss of conduction of motor, sensory and autonomic impulses although most or all the fibres may be in anatomical continuity. Recovery might therefore occur quite soon. It is difficult immediately after an injury to be certain of the extent of the injury although one can make a fairly informed guess on the basis of the nature of the injury. If, however, there has been complete interruption of the motor axons, within about 14 days there will be changes in the muscles' response to electrical stimuli which produce what used to be known as the 'reaction of degeneration'. It is now better described as alternation of the strength-duration curve. These changes indicate that there has been extensive damage to motor axons, that recovery at the best will be slow and that possibly the nerve has been completely divided. Of course immediately after an injury, there may be reasons for exploring the wound. For instance, there might be an open wound, an associated fracture or dislocation which requires an operation. A tendon may have been divided and obviously it is very important that, under these circumstances, if there is clinical evidence that the nerve has been divided, the surgeon should make a direct inspection of the nerve. If however, there is no indication for immediate operation, that is, if it is a closed injury, the wisest thing is to make a careful record of the clinical findings and wait. At the end of a fortnight the position is reviewed (see Chapter 4).

Injuries are not the only cause of lesions of peripheral nerves. There may be various diseases, metabolic disorders, infections or pressure from aneurysms, tumours, callus, scar tissue etc., which may lead to interruption of nerve conduction. As in so many other instances, in medicine and surgery, it is more important to think of the possibility of a diagnosis than to know very complicated tests. If one rapidly reviews in one's own mind the common causes of peripheral nerve lesions and considers whether they are applicable in the particular circumstances one will usually be able to make an accurate diagnosis. When one is reviewing causes, one can either start with the most frequent causes and consider or eliminate them in turn, or one can follow some consistent scheme such as considering causes in alphabetical order or taking them in groups according to age. Obviously, in different countries and in different ages the commonest causes will vary. The most likely diagnosis may well be different in a young child in England from an elderly man in Asia. For this reason it is more convenient to consider the various causes in the following groups.

Causes of peripheral nerve lesions

There are four main groups of causes of peripheral nerve lesions:
1 Trauma to the nerve
2 Pressure from adjacent structures
3 Diseases of the nerve or anterior horn cells
4 Ischaemia.

1 Trauma to the nerve

Trauma to the nerve may be considered under five headings:
(a) Concussion—temporary interruption of function, anatomical continuity.
(b) Contusion—temporary interruption of function and intraneural bruising which may lead to fibrosis.
(c) Division—complete division of all or some axon fibres and sheaths and the nerve sheath—usually due to a cut or high velocity missile.
(d) Stretching—disruption of some or all the nerve fibres and axon sheaths but usually pseudocontinuity of the main nerve sheath. Usually there is some intraneural haemorrhage. Later, there is entensive fibrosis. Recovery is never complete and often there is no useful recovery.
(e) Injections into a nerve.

In concussion and contusion, operation on the nerve is unnecessary. In stretching, no operation is effective. In division, operative repair is usually indicated.

2 Pressure from adjacent structures

Pressure on a nerve may be due to tumours, ganglia, bones, callus, fascial bands, aneurysm, haemorrhage, retraction during operations, splints or tourniquets. Removal of the compressing cause is nearly always required.

3   Diseases of the nerve or anterior horn cell

Diseases of the nerve:

(a)   Infections of the nerve, such as leprosy, or of the anterior horn cell, as in poliomyelitis and herpes.
(b)   Infections elsewhere in the body such as diphtheria, tuberculosis (producing amyloidosis) undulant fever.
(c)   Toxic agents, such as lead, arsenic and other chemicals.
(d)   Metabolic disorders such as in diabetes, uraemia, pulmonary neoplasms, vitamin deficiencies.
(e)   Ischaemic nerve lesions as in periateritis nodosa.
(f)   Peripheral neuropathy due to malignant disease, e.g. of the bronchus.

4   Ischaemia

As already explained, most peripheral nerves consist of a collection of nerve fibres or axons of which there are three main types:
(i)   Motor, i.e. fibres carrying efferent impulses to muscles.
(ii)   Sensory or afferent fibres conveying impulses from peripheral sensory end organs to the spinal cord. These are of many different types. The end organs may be situated in muscles (annulo spiral and flower spray) in tendons (Golgi organs), in joints or in the skin. Nerve fibres from muscles, tendons and joints control muscle activity and posture through a variety of reflex arcs. End organs in the skin are the media through which external stimuli reach the brain and produce sensations of heat, cold, touch, prick etc., and through which we are able to localize the site of a stimulus and discriminate differences in texture, two point discrimination, etc.
(iii)   Autonomic fibres, which control sweating, pilomotor activity, blood vessel tone and influence the metabolic activity of the region thus having a 'trophic' influence.

Complete division of a peripheral nerve produces flaccid paralysis of the muscles uniquely supplied by it, loss of sensation in the nerves' autonomous area, and loss of sweating, pilomotor activity and vasomotor control in the same area.

Diagnosis between permanent and temporary lesions is not easy, immediately after an injury, unless the nerve has been seen to be completely divided. In addition, anatomical variations may give the impression that a complete lesion is only partial. For instance, muscles may have a dual innervation or an anomalous nerve supply. Similarly, the area of skin supplied exclusively by a given peripheral nerve varies between individuals and with age. Examination of peripheral nerves depends on the patient's cooperation and, consciously or unconsciously, patients may appear to have anaesthetic areas or be unable to contract a muscle voluntarily. A fortnight after injury, certain signs can be elicited which indicate that the nerve endings in muscles have undergone degenerative changes. These are known as the 'reaction of degeneration' (q.v.) or altered strength duration curve. In addition, dryness of the skin and changes in skin texture indicate non-conduction in autonomic fibres whose distribution corresponds closely to the distribution of sensory fibres. Degeneration of sensory fibres also leads to loss of the axon reflex and alteration in the histamine response (q.v.). Further refinements in diagnostic techniques are the use of electro-myography and both motor and sensory nerve conduction times (q.v.).

Wallerian degeneration

If a nerve has been completely divided and the ends become separated, the nerve fibres distal to the lesion degenerate, leaving empty Schwann tubes (see Fig. 3.10). However, if a nerve suture is performed, the proximal nerve fibres (or axons) will grow into the empty tubes and ultimately lead to restoration of function (Fig. 3.11). Naturally, recovery is better in children in recent lesions, or in clean cuts; in elderly people, or in longstanding lesions, or where there has been extensive bruising or impairment of the blood supply to the nerve, the prognosis is worse.

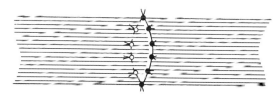

Fig. 3.11.   Nerve suture.

Lesions of the lumbar and sacral nerves

Intraspinal causes:

Injuries, dislocations, laminal fractures, disc protrusions, tumours, and congenital anomalies may all cause interference with function of the nerves of the cauda equina. This can vary in degree from one extreme, complete loss of motor function and sensation in the legs and 'saddle area' with loss of bladder and bowel control, to the other extreme, of severe pain referred to the distribution of one segment with minimal motor and sensory changes.

In the latter case there is often associated spasm of the back muscles with scoliosis, stiffness and limitation of straight leg raising.

The common neurological signs of a disc lesion are (1) weakness of the extensor hallucis longus (L5 lesion), (2) loss or diminution of the ankle jerk (S1 lesion), (3) impairment of sensation in the relevant body segment.

Treatment is firstly, to diagnose the cause and secondly, to remove the cause either by conservative means or operation.

One special form of cauda equina lesion should be mentioned, i.e. intermittent claudication symptoms or pain in the buttocks, thighs and calves on exercise, unassociated with peripheral vascular disease, but due to spinal stenosis. Central vascular disease may play a part in this.

Femoral nerve lesions

The femoral nerve is branch of the lumbar plexus. It is formed by roots formed from the second, third and fourth lumbar spinal nerves. To reach the anterior area of the thigh the nerve passes through the iliac fossa from the lumbar plexus, near the lumbar vertebrae, to the posterior surface of the inguinal ligament and into the groin and thigh. It then forms the following branches:

MOTOR:
(a)   Sartorius muscle
(b)   Quadriceps femoris muscle
(c)   Pectineus muscles

CUTANEOUS:
(a)   Intermediate cutaneous nerve to the skin on the front of the thigh
(b)   Medial cutaneous nerve to the skin on the medial surface of the thigh
(c)   Saphenous nerve to the medial side of the leg ankle and foot

Lesions of the femoral nerve cause paralysis of the quadriceps and loss of sensation on the front of the thigh. They may be due to injuries, e.g. knife or bullet wounds, injury at operation, aneurysms or they may be associated with haemorrhage into the ilio-psoas muscle in conditions such as haemophilia.

Pressure on the femoral nerve can usually be removed, but operative repair of a severed femoral nerve is nearly always impossible. If the weak or paralysed quadriceps causes collapse of the patient's knee,
1   he can wear a jointed caliper.
2   the hamstring muscles can be transplanted into the patella or lower end of the femur.

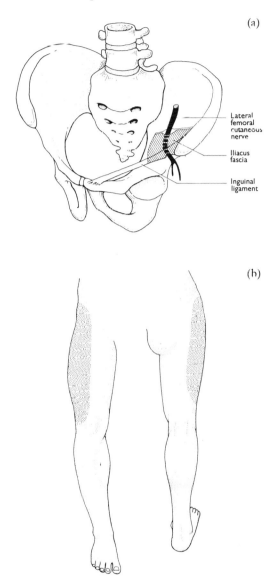

Fig. 3.12. (a) The lateral femoral cutaneous nerve. (b) Areas supplied by the nerve.

3   he may be able to walk normally with functioning glutei and calf muscles, provided there is no flexion deformity of the knee. If a flexion deformity is present, it must be corrected by either division, elongation or transplantation of the hamstring muscles and gastrocnemius and joint capsule. If this is not enough, by a corrective supracondylar osteotomy of the femur.

Lesions of the lateral femoral cutaneous nerve of the thigh

This could be considered as the cutaneous branch of the femoral nerve. It is formed, at the lumbar plexus from spinal nerves Lumbar 2 and 3. It enters the lateral surface of the thigh near the anterior superior iliac spine after passing behind the inguinal ligament to leave the abdominal cavity. The nerve is superficial to the skin of the thigh and gives cutaneous nerves to the lateral surface of the thigh to the level of the knee.

Lateral femoral cutaneous lesions

This nerve may be compressed either in the abdomen by fat or as it passes through the abdominal wall (Fig. 3.12). The symptoms are burning pain and impairment of sensation on the antero-lateral aspect of the thigh. The treatment is weight reduction; occasionally decompression as it passes through the inguinal ligament is indicated. Minor examples of this lesion may be produced by tight clothing, belts, corsets, etc.

Lesions of the obturator nerve (Fig. 3.13)

This is formed by roots from Lumbar spinal nerves numbers 2, 3 and 4. It arises at the side of the certebral column within the psoas muscle. The nerve then enters the true pelvis to pass forwards and out of the pelvic cavity via the obturator foramen at its anterior and superior aspect. It enters the thigh to form the anterior superficial and posterior deep divisions. The functions of these divisons are:

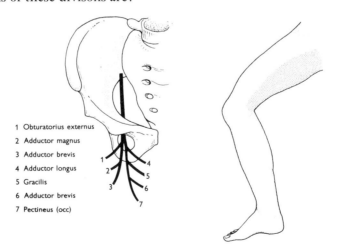

1 Obturatorius externus
2 Adductor magnus
3 Adductor brevis
4 Adductor longus
5 Gracilis
6 Adductor brevis
7 Pectineus (occ)

Fig. 3.13.   The obturator nerve.

Anterior superficial

Branches to

(a) The hip joint
(b) Obturator externus muscle
(c) Adductor longus muscle
(d) Gracilis muscle

Posterior deep

Branches to

(a) Obturator externus muscle
(b) Adductor brevis
(c) Adductor magnus muscle
(d) The knee joint

It may also serve:

(e) Pectineus muscle
(f) Adductor brevis muscle

Obturator nerve lesions classically occur in association with an obturator hernia. The symptoms are pain in the adductor region and weakness of the adductors.

The treatment is removal of the hernia.

The sciatic nerve

The sciatic trunk (which is a better name for this nerve) is a large collection of nerve fibres providing most of the nerve supply to the lower limb. It is formed from the sacral plexus which has nerve roots formed by the anterior primary rami of Lumbar 4 and 5 and Sacral 1, 2 and 3 spinal nerves.

As the sacral plexus is formed on the anterior surface of the sacrum, the sciatic trunk on its path to the leg must pass out of the bony pelvis; it emerges from the pelvis via the greater sciatic foramen on the postero-lateral surface of the pelvis. (Fig. 3.14).

The sciatic trunk is oval in section and is about 2 centimetres wide. It is formed of two main divisions combined within one sheath. In some people these are divided at pelvic level and the two parts are separated from the pelvis downwards. This is called 'high division'.

After the nerve leaves the pelvis it is situated about midway between the ischial tuberosity (upon which the trunk rests in sitting) and the great trochanter of the femur.

The nerve passes down through the tissues on the posterior thigh to the level of the popliteal space which is behind the knee. It supplies the hamstring muscles en route. At some point in the lower half of the thigh the nerve bifurcates into the medial popliteal and common peroneal nerves which are the main nerves supplying the limb from this division distally (Fig. 3.15).

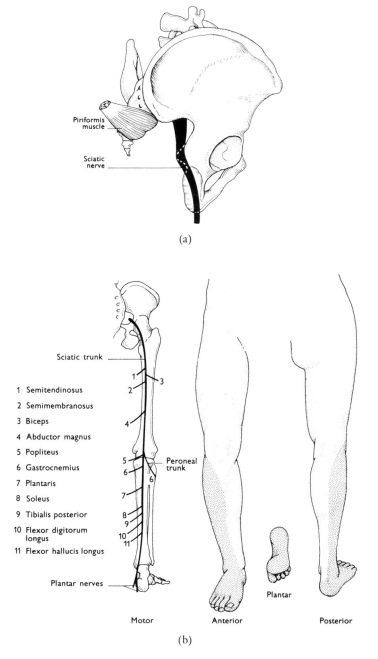

(a)

1 Semitendinosus
2 Semimembranosus
3 Biceps
4 Abductor magnus
5 Popliteus
6 Gastrocnemius
7 Plantaris
8 Soleus
9 Tibialis posterior
10 Flexor digitorum longus
11 Flexor hallucis longus

Sciatic trunk

Peroneal trunk

Plantar nerves

Motor   Anterior   Plantar   Posterior

(b)

Fig. 3.14. (a) The sacral plexus related to the sciatic notch. (b) The sciatic nerve relating to the areas it supplies.

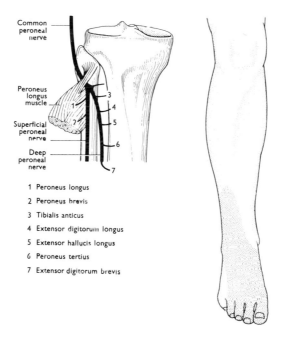

Common peroneal nerve

Peroneus longus muscle

Superficial peroneal nerve

Deep peroneal nerve

1 Peroneus longus

2 Peroneus brevis

3 Tibialis anticus

4 Extensor digitorum longus

5 Extensor hallucis longus

6 Peroneus tertius

7 Extensor digitorum brevis

Fig. 3.15. The common peroneal nerve relating to the areas it supplies.

Sciatic nerve lesions

Complete sciatic nerve lesions are seen as a result of buttock and thigh wounds, injections into the nerve, dislocations of the hip and occasionally tumours, such as neurofibromata. The signs are paralysis and loss of sensation below the knee. If the nerve does not recover, ulceration of the sole of the foot, infection and trophic changes are likely to occur, and ultimately, a below-knee amputation is usually needed. Operations such as arthrodesis of the foot are contra-indicated. Special boots and insoles and below-knee irons are usually helpful in the interim period.

The medial popliteal nerve

This nerve is the larger of the two bifurcations of the sciatic nerve. It continues on distally from the popliteal space (posterior to the knee) to the middle of the calf.

It supplies articular branches to the knee joint and muscular branches to the gastrocnemius, soleus and the popliteus muscles. The cutaneous branch supplies skin on the upper calf.

Medial popliteal nerve lesions

A lesion of this nerve gives the patient anaesthesia of the sole of the foot and paralysis of the muscles which are attached to tendo-calcaneous resulting in a calcaneo-carus deformity. Little can be done except to provide a well-padded insole and instruct the patient to examine the sole of his foot with a mirror each day.

The posterior tibial nerve

This nerve is the distal continuation of the medial popliteal nerve which passes down to the medial side of the ankle to the sole of the foot. Its position in relation to the ankle is midway between the heel and the medial malleolus. In the sole of the foot it becomes the medial and lateral plantar nerves. The nerve supplies muscular branches to the soleus muscle, tibialis posterior muscle, flexor digitorum muscle, and the flexor hallucis longus muscle. It also gives off cutaneous branches to the skin of the heel and hind-part of the sole of the foot.

Posterior tibial nerve lesions

These lesions are characterized by anaesthesia of the heel and sole of the foot and paralysis of the intrinsic muscles of the foot leading to a pes-cavus deformity. The treatment is usually the provision of a special insole.

The digital nerves

The plantar nerves, derived from the posterior tibial nerve, supply the four plantar digital nerves to the toes. These nerves supply articular branches to the joints and muscular branches to the intrinsic muscles of the foot.

Digital nerve lesions

The commonest lesion is a 'neuroma' of the nerve supplying the third and fourth toes. The patient complains of severe intermittent pain on walking and the treatment is excision of the neuroma.

The common peroneal nerve

The common peroneal (Fig. 3.15) nerve is the lesser division of the sciatic trunk. It is formed in the sacral plexus from spinal nerves Lumbar

4 and 5 and Sacral 1 and 2. From the posterior lower third of the thigh the nerve passes laterally and is superficial as it winds around the head and neck of the fibula where it can be felt by the fingers and is vulnerable to trauma and pressure from splintage or bandaging.

It becomes (a) the anterior tibial nerve and (b) the peroneal nerve. (a) The *anterior tibial nerve* (Fig. 3.16) passes distally to the anterior surface of the ankle joint. Within the superior surface of the foot it bifurcates into the medial and lateral terminal branches.

Branches:

(a)   As the anterior tibial nerve:
1 extensor digitorum longus muscle; 2 peroneus tertius muscle; 3 extensor hallucis longus muscle; 4 tibialis anterior muscle.

(b)   As the *lateral terminal branch* in the foot.
1 extensor digitorum brevis muscle; 2 the tarsal joints; 3 the metatarsal joints.

(c)   As the *medial terminal branch* in the foot:
It supplies the skin on adjacent sides of the great toe and second toe (Fig. 3.19a).

(d)   *The peroneal nerve*
This is a division of the common peroneal nerve which first serves the peroneus longus and brevis muscles and then becomes a cutaneous nerve which divides into branches which serve the skin over the upper surface of the foot. (Fig. 3.17).

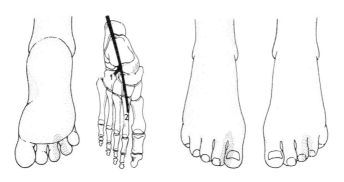

1 Extensor digitorum brevis   Sensory distribution
2 1st dorsal interosseus

Motor distribution

Fig. 3.16.   The cutaneous sensory area on the foot supplied by the anterior tibial nerve.

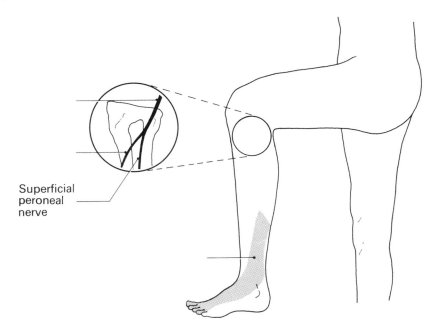

Fig. 3.17. The cutaneous sensory area on the foot served by the peroneal nerve.

Common peroneal lesions

The patient suffers from 'foot-drop', i.e. inability to dorsiflex or evert the foot and toes and there is impairment of sensation on the dorsum of the foot and antero-lateral aspect of the shin (see Fig. 3.19b). If the nerve lesion is irrecoverable the patient can either wear an iron and toe-spring or alternatively the tibialis posterior muscle may be transplanted through the interosseous membrane to the front of the leg and dorsum of the foot.

Splintage for peripheral nerve lesions

The splints supplied to patients with these conditions must be as unobtrusive and as light in weight as possible. They are supplied for a variety of reasons:

1   As 'lively' splints. These are spring loaded devices (Fig. 3.18) which oppose the action of unparalysed muscles. The patient contracts his unaffected muscles against the springs to exercise the muscles and prevent stiffness and deformity of the joints. They also act as partial functional substitutes for the paralysed muscles.

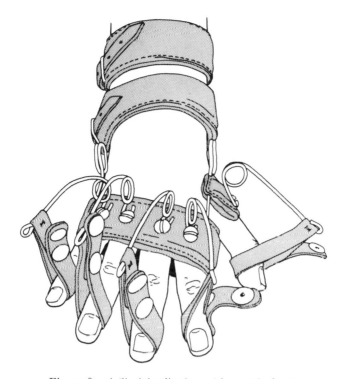

Fig. 3.18. A 'lively' splint in position on the hand.

2   To maintain the limb in an acceptable and usable position. For example, if the patient has a dropped wrist, a 'cock-up' splint may be supplied to hold the hand in a position which will enable the patient to hold a writing or eating utensil (see Fig. 3.19a and b).

3   To hold the limb in the 'optimum position of rest' so that the paralysed muscles are not stretched and the unparalysed muscles do not become contracted. Stretched denervated muscles may undergo irrecoverable changes.

Splintage for peripheral nerve lesions of the lower limb

Damage to the common peroneal (lateral popliteal) nerve. In the lower limb this is the lesion most likely to require splintage. This nerve is the lateral half of the sciatic nerve: it first passes down in the posterior thigh. It then leaves the sciatic trunk to wind around the neck of the fibula where it can be rolled against the bone with one's finger. It then passes forwards to supply the muscles which lift the forefoot and extend (dorsiflex) the toes. When the nerve is damaged the forefoot hangs down, and the toes catch in

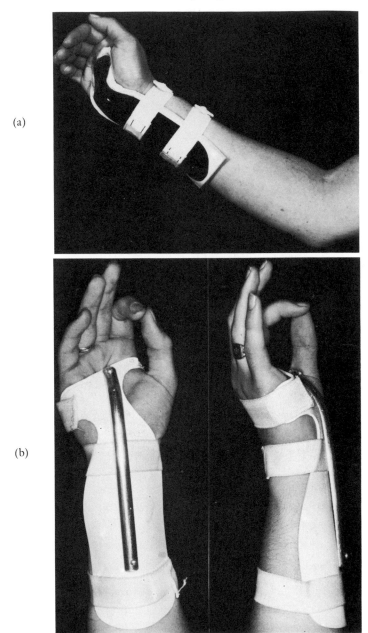

(a)

(b)

Fig. 3.19. (a) A cock-up splint in position. (b) Another form of the cock-up splint.

the ground when walking. The following splints are available for use in the conservative treatment of the deformity:

RIZZOLI SPLINT (Fig. 3.20)

This is a strong, flat spring which passes down the posterior surface of the leg to be inserted into the leather of the back of the patient's shoe. The upper end of the spring is attached to a metal band which passes round the calf. The splint is covered in flesh-coloured material to make it as unobtrusive as possible. Once the spring is applied and the shoe is laced up, the foot is held in a corrected position and does not hang down in walking.

This splint is only for use on patients with paralysis of the anterior muscles of the leg. When the posterior muscles are paralysed, the spring and band would compress the back of the leg and cause a splint sore.

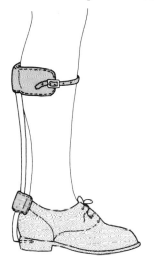
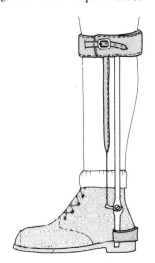

Fig. 3.20.   A Rizzoli splint in position.   Fig. 3.21.   Drop-foot springs.

DROP-FOOT SPRINGS

(Fig. 3.21). These serve a similar function as the Rizzoli splint but are more obtrusive. The hinged bar of the splint passes down the side of the leg to be inserted into a socket in the heel of the shoe. The hinge is spring-loaded and the strength of the spring can be varied to meet the needs of the patient. It is functionally efficient but aesthetically unacceptable to girls.

TOE-RAISING SPRINGS

A modified shoe can also be used for patients with a drop-foot deformity. (Fig. 3.22). These are easily seen on the patient. The spring forms a right-angled triangle with the foot and the leg. The upper end of the spring is attached to a band around the leg below the knee; the lower end is inserted into the upper surface of the toe end of the shoe. The spring serves to lift the front end of the shoe and thus the foot. The band around the leg tends

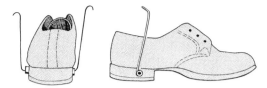

Fig. 3.22.   A modified shoe for a patient with a drop-foot deformity with inserts for a double below knee iron.

to slip down; if this happens the spring becomes ineffective. If the band is tightened to prevent it slipping, it may cause pain and oedema of the foot. (Fig. 3.23).

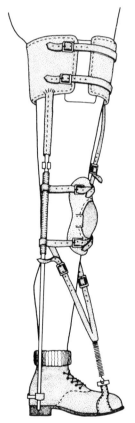

Fig. 3.23.   Toe-raising spring.

Complete paralysis of the lower leg and foot

The leg below the knee is supplied by two main nerves; the common peroneal (lateral popliteal) and the medial popliteal nerves. If both are affected by a lesion, the leg and foot are flail; the foot is unstable when it is placed on the ground, for example, to support the body in standing or walking. The ankle and foot must therefore be stabilized so that the foot is 'plantigrade' and the leg is vertical—that is, so that it provides a stable platform upon which the patient can stand. In some instances this can be done surgically; if splintage is to be used, however, it must be functional rather than elegant; it must have sufficient strength to withstand a heavy work load.

DOUBLE BELOW-KNEE IRONS (Fig. 3.24)

These are two parallel bars which pass down on either side of the lower leg. At the top of the splint they are attached to a supporting band which passes around the leg; at the lower end they are bent and inserted into rectangular sockets placed on either side of the heel of the patient's shoe. The shoe must be adapted when the splint is ordered. A strap passes from one bar to the other behind the leg at the level of the malleoli, to hold the bars in their sockets in the shoe. Whilst the patient is wearing this splint no dorsiflexion or plantarflexion of the ankle joint or foot is possible. Alternatively round sockets may be used with anterior and/or posterior stops which allow limited ankle motion (Fig. 3.25).

SINGLE BELOW-KNEE IRON WITH T-STRAP (Fig. 3.26)

A single iron bar passes down on one side of the leg. It is attached at the upper end to a supporting band around the leg below the knee. At its lower end it is bent and inserted into a socket in the heel of the shoe (Fig. 3.24). The shape of the socket may be:

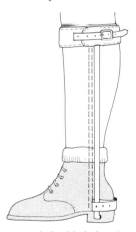

Fig. 3.24.   A double below-knee iron.

1   Rectangular when the bar entering the socket is also rectangular. Thus no dorsiflexion or plantarflexion is possible whilst the splint is being worn or,

2   Circular with a cylindrical shape of bar to enter the socket. Thus plantarflexion or dorsiflexion are permitted when this splint is worn. However, a metal 'stop' on the shoe may be fitted. If this is in front of the bar dorsiflexion is prevented; should it be placed behind the bar plantarflexion is prevented.

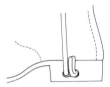

Fig. 3.25.   A circular socket with stop inserted into the heel of a shoe.

T-STRAPS

These are straps which are attached to the gusset of the shoe. The cross-bar of the T-shape fits around the ankle and over the below-knee iron. It is used to correct an inversion or eversion deformity of the foot.

CORRECTING INVERSION OF THE FOOT

Inversion is a deformity which is present when the sole of the foot is turned inwards towards the median line. To avoid inversion, the patient is supplied with an inside iron and an outside T-strap.

CORRECTING EVERSION OF THE FOOT

Eversion exists when the foot is deformed with the sole of the foot turned away from the midline and facing towards the lateral surface. It may be looked on as an extreme example of flat foot.

An outside iron and an inside T-strap are used to counter excessive eversion (Fig. 3.26).

Lesions affecting the brachial plexus

Relevant anatomy

The nerve supply to the upper extremity is the brachial plexus. This consists of an extensive grouping of nerve roots at the cervical region of the spinal cord and spinal column. The nerve roots then form large cords

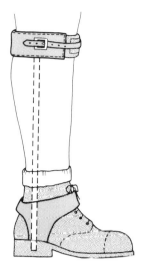

Fig. 3.26. An outside iron and inside 'T' strap.

of nerve tissue and their branches which pass through the shoulder from the neck down to the axilla. It has the following important relations:

1   *The clavicle.* This bone passes across the middle of the brachial plexus on its anterior surface. Severe complicated fractures of the clavicle may result in a brachial plexus lesion.

2   *The scapula.* The brachial plexus is related to the anterior surface of the bone and, again, severe complicated fractures of the bone may involve the plexus.

3   *The shoulder joint.* The brachial plexus is adjacent and dislocations of the joint may involve the plexus.

4   *The axillary artery.* The three cords of the brachial plexus are in direct relationship to this artery.

Although lesions of the spinal cord usually affect the 'long tracts' producing upper motor neurone paralysis or spastic paralysis, certain vascular lesions of the cervical spine (e.g. the anterior spinal artery syndrome) may cause destruction of anterior horn cells thus producing a lower motor neurone type of paralysis with flaccidity and muscle wasting. Although this is not literally a brachial plexus lesion it may mimic peripheral lesions so closely that it is convenient to describe this syndrome in association with brachial plexus lesions. Similarly, certain virus infections affecting the anterior horn cells, (poliomyelitis, herpes, amyotrophic myalgia) often produce widespread flaccid paralysis resembling in some respects, lesions of the brachial plexus. At a slightly more peripheral site both motor and sensory nerve roots may be affected by protruding disc material, tumours

or osteophytes, occluding the intervertebral foramina, and unilateral dislocations of the cervical spine frequently compress one cervical nerve root.

The classical brachial plexus lesion is a supraclavicular traction injury
resulting from violent separation of the shoulder from the neck, it is often
associated with a head injury and may be partial or complete. If the injury
is a violent one the lesion is usually permanent and may extend centrally
as far as the nerve roots and even affect the spinal cord. Lesions of the lower
roots are frequently associated with damage to the cervical sympathetic
chain producing a 'Horner's syndrome'. At a still more peripheral level
direct violence to the clavicle may occasionally damage the underlying
brachial plexus. Below the clavicle, damage to the brachial plexus may
result either from a dislocation or from a fracture dislocation of the shoulder,
indeed, a displaced head of humerus may cause permanent pressure on the
plexus.

Penetrating injuries such as gunshot wounds and stab wounds may
cause lesions at any level and are often associated with vascular injuries.
We have, therefore, a large variety of causes of brachial plexus lesions and
a considerable number of different syndromes; it is proposed to describe
briefly, the most frequently encountered syndromes and their commoner
causes.

Lesions of the main branches of the brachial plexus

Lesions of the nerve to the serratus anterior muscle

(a) *The serratus anterior muscle.* This muscle is superficial and is easily
seen on the lateral surface of the thorax. It is a sheet of muscle tissue which is
attached by finger-like projections to eight upper ribs. It converges to be
attached at its medial end to the vertebral border of the scapula. Thus it is
situated between the thorax and scapula.

Functions of the muscle
This muscle is one of the controlling muscles of the scapula, it acts in
all movements which occur at the shoulder when the arm is raised. The
scapula moves freely over the posterior surface of the thorax, and would
without the serratus anterior 'wing' away from it. When the humerus or
clavicle are moved the serratus anterior muscle assists these movements.
(b) *The nerve to the serratus anterior muscle:* This arises, in the brachial
plexus (Fig. 3.6) from the posterior trunks of the cervical 5, 6 and 7 spinal
nerve roots. From the plexus, it passes over the outer border of the first rib.

After it crosses the first rib it passes down the side of the rib cage to supply the muscle on its exterior surface.

Serratus anterior nerve lesions

This nerve can be injured either by pressure on the side of the neck as in carrying a heavy load or in the course of a thoracotomy or excision of breast operation; it is also liable to suffer virus infections. The result is paralysis of the serratus anterior muscle, i.e. the vertebral border of the scapula sticks out (winged scapula) especially when the patient tries to raise his arm or push against an object. In the case of virus infections the ultimate prognosis is usually good in time but recovery may take two years. Occasionally the permanent disability is so great as to justify anchoring the scapula to the chest wall.

Relevant anatomy

The suprascapular nerve

The stability of the ball and socket joints, the shoulder and hip joints, depends upon groups of muscle with the important function of ensuring that the ball is always in the socket no matter what the position of the bone attached to the ball. In the relatively shallow socket of the glenoid cavity this function is important. The muscles, in addition to being prime movers

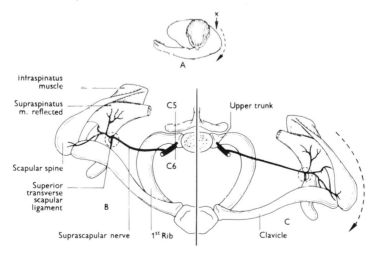

Fig. 3.27. The suprascapular nerve—superior aspect.

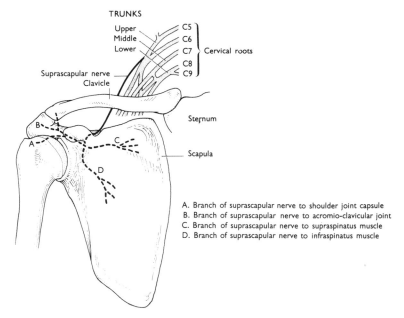

TRUNKS

Upper
Middle
Lower

C5
C6
C7 } Cervical roots
C8
C9

Suprascapular nerve
Clavicle

Sternum

Scapula

A. Branch of suprascapular nerve to shoulder joint capsule
B. Branch of suprascapular nerve to acromio-clavicular joint
C. Branch of suprascapular nerve to supraspinatus muscle
D. Branch of suprascapular nerve to infraspinatus muscle

Fig. 3.28.   Suprascapular nerve and its branches.

which initiate a particular movement, also pull the head of the humerus towards the glenoid cavity by contracting whenever a new position is adopted. Such a group of muscles surrounds the shoulder joint and the suprascapular nerve supplies two of the muscles which support the shoulder capsule. They are called the supraspinatus and infraspinatus muscles.

The suprascapular nerve leaves the upper trunk of the brachial plexus and passes backwards to pass through the suprascapular notch which is on the superior border of the scapula (Fig. 3.28).

Suprascapular nerve lesions

Apart from virus infections this nerve may suffer from indirect trauma. The result is inability to initiate abduction of the arm and difficulty in controlling scapulo-humeral movement in the middle ranges. The patient can usually hold his arm vertically up if helped to get it there. On attempting to lower the arm slowly it falls suddenly—this is similar to the torn supraspinatus syndrome (q.v.).

No specific treatment is possible, in time the patient learns various trick movements which lessens the disability. A number of muscle transplant operations have been devised but these are not very successful. Very occasionally the disability is bad enough to justify an arthrodesis of the shoulder.

Lesions of the muscle-cutaneous nerve

Injuries to the nerve, to the biceps brachii and coraco-brachialis muscles are rare but the nerve may be involved as part of a virus infection of the brachial plexus. Specific remedial measures are not usually necessary as the condition recovers in time.

Lesions affecting the ulnar nerve

This nerve is formed in the lower part of the brachial plexus mainly from nerve roots formed by the eight cervical and first thoracic spinal nerves. After passing down the upper arm on its medial side it passes behind the prominent medial epicondyle, which has a sulcus, or groove, in which the nerve rests. The nerve is superficial at this point and is often hurt when the medial epicondyle is knocked (the 'funny' bone).

From this point it passes into the medial side of the forearm and enters the hand on the medial side of the ulnar artery after crossing the flexor retinaculum (Fig. 3.29).

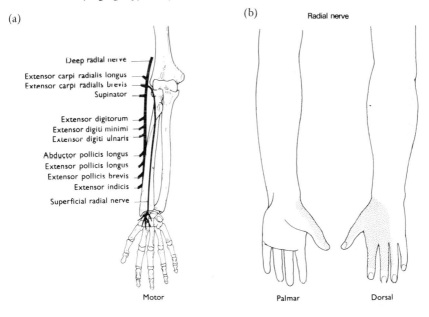

Fig. 3.29. (a) The radial nerve. (b) The sensory supply of the radial nerve to the hand.

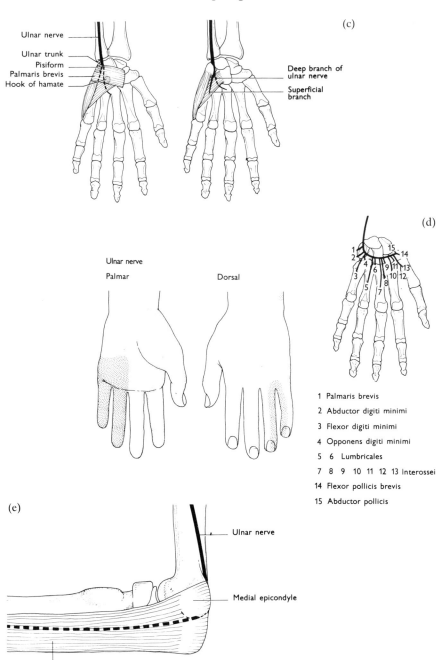

(c)

Ulnar nerve
Ulnar trunk
Pisiform
Palmaris brevis
Hook of hamate

Deep branch of
ulnar nerve
Superficial
branch

Ulnar nerve

Palmar   Dorsal

(d)

1 Palmaris brevis

2 Abductor digiti minimi

3 Flexor digiti minimi

4 Opponens digiti minimi

5   6 Lumbricales

7 8 9 10 11 12 13 Interossei

14 Flexor pollicis brevis

15 Abductor pollicis

(e)

Ulnar nerve

Medial epicondyle

Forearm flexor group

Fig. 3.29. (c–e) The ulnar nerves, its branches and the areas it supplies.

MAIN BRANCHES OF THE ULNAR NERVE:

1   *in the forearm :*

(a)   The flexor carpi ulnaris muscle.

(b)   flexor digitorum profundus muscle.

2   *in the wrist and hand :*

(a)   a palmar cutaneous branch to the medial side of the wrist and hand.

(b)   the palmaris brevis muscle.

(c)   cutaneous supply to the skin of the little finger and medial half of the ring finger.

(d)   the interosseous muscles situated between the metacarpal bones.

(e)   the muscles in the hypothenar eminence.

(f)   the medial lumbrical muscles.

(g)   the adductor pollicis longus muscle.

Ulnar nerve lesions

The ulnar nerve supplies the small muscles of the hand and sensation to the little finger and ulnar border of the hand. Lack of the latter deprives us of an important sensory element and guide in performing actions such as writing when we rest our little finger or hand on the paper.

Paralysis of the small muscles impairs pinch and fine movements more than grip—if untreated it may lead to a 'claw hand' (q.v.).

Lesions of the ulnar nerve commonly occur in leprosy. Pressure on the ulnar nerve may be produced by a band of fascia at the elbow, i.e. the thickened proximal edge of the fascia joining the two heads of the flexor carpi ulnaris. Commonly this is a sequel of cubitus valgus due to an injury to the lower end of the humerus in childhood.

Lesions of the ulnar nerve may occur at the wrist from cuts or wounds and in the palm of the hand from pressure from a ganglion.

Treatment is to remove the cause of the pressure and suture the nerve if it has been divided.

The median nerve

This nerve is formed in the brachial plexus of roots from spinal nerves cervical five, six, seven and eight and thoracic one. It passes down the upper arm to the area above the elbow joint where it is closely related to the brachial artery and the anterior surface of humerus. It enters the forearm approximately at the centre point of the elbow joint and passes centrally down the forearm to the centre of the wrist. Shortly after entering the fore-

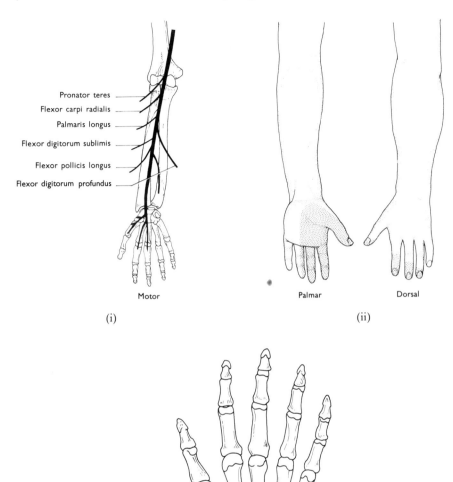

Pronator teres

Flexor carpi radialis

Palmaris longus

Flexor digitorum sublimis

Flexor pollicis longus

Flexor digitorum profundus

Motor

(i)

Palmar   Dorsal

(ii)

Opponens branch

Median nerve

(iii)

Fig. 3.30. The median nerve, at elbow and the sensory areas it supplies. (i) Median nerve. (ii) Cutaneous supply of the nerve to the hand. (iii) Median nerve at wrist.

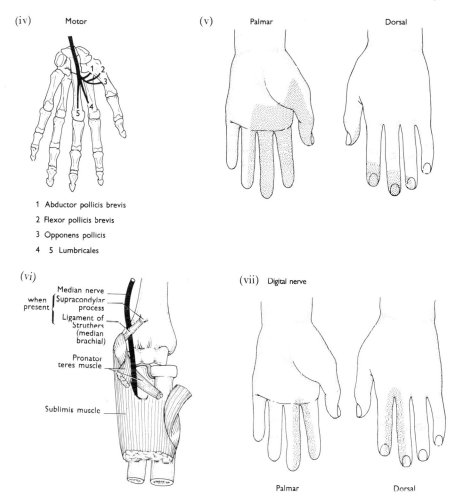

(iv) Motor

1 Abductor pollicis brevis

2 Flexor pollicis brevis

3 Opponens pollicis

4 5 Lumbricales

(v) Palmar   Dorsal

(vi)

Median nerve

when Supracondylar
present process

Ligament of
Struthers
(median
brachial)

Pronator
teres muscle

Sublimis muscle

(vii) Digital nerve

Palmar   Dorsal

Fig. 3.30. (iv) Median nerve in hand (v) Sensory distribution of the median nerve
in the hand.

arm it gives off a branch called the anterior interosseous nerve. At the wrist
the nerve enters the anterior of the hand under the flexor retinaculum which
helps to form the 'carpal tunnel'; this is a compartment with mainly bony
boundaries. In the hand it gives off a muscular branch which supplies three
of the muscles in the thenar eminence, called abductor pollicis brevis,
opponens pollicis and flexor pollicis brevis. It also gives five digital palmar
cutaneous branches which supply the anterior of the lateral two and one-
half fingers and the thumb (Fig. 3.30).

Median nerve lesions

Affections of the median nerve are common and very important. Loss of sensation in the thumb and index and middle fingers deprives the hand of its most skilled function—the 'eyes' at the ends of these digits which give us vital information about the objects we are handling. In addition, paralysis of the thumb muscles deprives us of adequate power of opposition and pinch. Furthermore, causalgia (spontaneous pain, q.v.) is not uncommon with lesions of the median nerve. Although the median nerve may be affected by virus infections and periarteritis nodosa the commonest median nerve lesions are described below:

The carpal tunnel syndrome

This is commonly seen in middle-aged women. It may be associated with tenosynovitis of the flexor tendons including tuberculous and rheumatoid tendon sheath infection.

Classically the patient complains of burning pain at night in the distribution of the median nerve. There may be wasting of the thenar muscles and impairment of fine sensation in the thumb and index finger. The best test for this is recognition of embossed letters with the eyes closed. In doubtful cases estimation of nerve conduction times are useful as delay in conduction (diminished velocity) at the wrist indicates compression at this site. Mild symptoms may be relieved by splinting the wrist in slight flexion, but if the symptoms return after removing the splint the minor procedure of division of the transverse carpal ligament will produce a permanent cure, provided the whole of the ligament is divided—and it extends distally into the palm of the hand to merge with the palmar fascia.

Division (partial or complete) of the median nerve commonly occurs with cuts at the wrist. There is often also division of flexor tendons and the ulnar nerve. There will be loss of sensation and sweating in the median area and paralysis and wasting of the ball of the thumb. The treatment is repair of the nerve. If there are associated tendon injuries these should be repaired first and the ends of the median nerve placed in a silastic tube. Some six weeks after injury, the nerve is exposed, the silastic tube removed and formal nerve suture performed. Even if there are no other injuries it is usually wise to suture the skin, place the nerve ends in a silastic tube and perform a formal suture one month later. The median nerve may also be damaged at the wrist by a dislocation of the lunate bone.

Injuries to the median nerve at a higher level will cause more extensive motor weakness, e.g. flexors of the thumb and fingers and weakness of pronation. In the forearm there is usually associated damage to muscles and of course the median nerve function may be impaired in Volkmann's ischaemic contracture when the blood supply to the forearm muscles is impaired, e.g. by a supracondylar fracture.

Damage to the median nerve at the elbow may occur from an elbow dislocation, injections of noxious drugs or cuts or wounds. The brachial artery may be damaged as well and the median nerve has been damaged in the course of operation to ligature the brachial artery.

The circumflex nerve

This nerve arises from the brachial plexus and passes backwards through a space formed by muscles, tendons and the humerus. It is in intimate contact with the surgical neck of the humerus as it winds around the humerus and therefore is vulnerable in fractures of the surgical neck of the humerus. The nerve supplies: (a) the deltoid muscle; (b) the teres minor muscle; (c) the capsule of the shoulder joint; (d) an area of skin over the point of the shoulder.

Circumflex nerve lesions

This nerve may be injured when the shoulder is dislocated. Although the deltoid muscle is paralysed the disability is usually surprisingly small provided the other shoulder muscles and particularly the spinati are active. Treatment is by physiotherapy and active use; the prognosis for ultimate recovery after nine to eighteen months is good. The circumflex nerve may also be involved in so-called myalgic amyotrophy which is generally believed to be a virus infection. The ultimate prognosis is good.

Lesions affecting the radial nerve

This is the largest branch of the brachial plexus. It arises from the posterior cord of the brachial plexus, enters the axilla and then winds around the posterior and lateral aspects of the humerus in a long spiral extending nearly the length of the bone. There is a groove on the humerus, the musculo-spiral groove into which the nerve fits on its passage down the arm. At the end of its spiral it may be felt in front of the lateral condyle of the humerus before it enters the lateral side of the forearm. In this region the nerve gives off a branch, the posterior interosseous nerve, and then passes down the anterior upper two-thirds of the forearm. About the lower third of the forearm it winds towards the posterior aspect of the thumb and

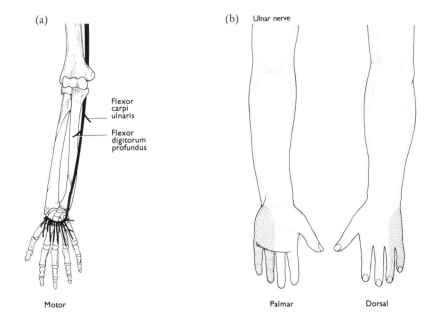

The ulnar nerve and the sensory areas it supplies.

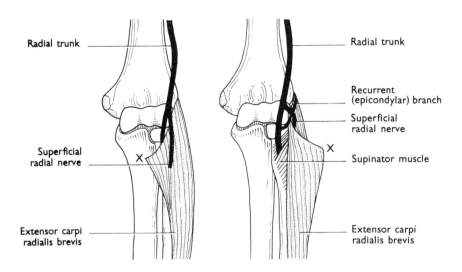

X is attachment to fascia of forearm flexor group

Fig. 3.31. The radial nerve, its branches and the sensory areas it supplies.

forms its two terminating lateral and medial digital branches. The lateral digital nerve serves the pad of the thumb and the medial branch supplies four digital nerves which are cutaneous branches to the skin of the posterior surface of the lateral two and a half fingers (Fig. 3.31).

MAIN BRANCHES:
In the upper arm:
(a) the triceps muscle; (b) the brachio-radialis muscle; (c) the extensor carpi radialis longus muscle; (d) the anconeus muscle; (e) part of the brachialis muscle.

In the forearm:
as the posterior interosseous nerve
(a) the extensor carpi radialis brevis muscle; (b) the extensor pollicis longus muscle; (c) the supinator muscle; (d) the extensor digitorum muscle; (e) the extensor digiti minimi muscle; (f) the extensor carpi ulnaris muscle; (g) the extensor pollicis longus muscle; (h) the abductor pollicis longus muscle; (i) the extensor indicis muscle; (j) the extensor pollicis brevis muscle; (k) the carpal joints and ligaments.

These muscles are mainly involved in extension, as the names of most of them indicate. Thus they contribute to extension of the elbow, extension of the wrist and extension and abduction of the thumb.

Radial nerve lesions

This nerve may be damaged by pressure in the axilla (as from a crutch or chair back) by a fracture of the shaft of the humerus, and fractures or dislocations involving the elbow. It may also be damaged by a tourniquet or in the course of operations on the humerus, elbow or head of radius. In the majority of closed lesions spontaneous recovery will occur but in open lesions, e.g. due to cuts or wounds the nerve can be divided. Occasionally callus formation or scarring cause loss of function. The treatment is:
1   To prevent overstretching of paralysed muscles and the development of contractures.
2   To release the nerve from pressure.
3   To suture the nerve if it has been divided.
4   To perform a tendon transplant operation if the nerve is irrecoverable.

The classical procedure is to transplant the pronator teres muscle into the extensor carpi radialis muscle, the palmaris longus muscle into the extensor pollicis longus muscle and the flexor carpi ulnaris muscle into the extensor digitorus muscle.

Hand and finger deformities in paralysed patients

Following paralysis of the intrinsic muscles, i.e. the lumbricals and interossei what is known as a claw hand, may develop. Essentially this consists of hyperextension of the metacarpo-phalangeal joints and flexion of the interphalangeal joints. If neglected, such deformities may ultimately become fixed and the joint capsules become fibrosed in the deformed position.

The cause of this deformity is a disturbance of the balance between flexor and extensor muscle at each joint.

Muscle and tendon transfers in paralysis

Under certain circumstances, where one group of muscles are weak, it is possible to transfer the muscles and tendons of another group as a substitute. It is important that the muscle to be transferred should be:

1   Strong and active enough for its new function.
2   Able to be re-educated to perform a new movement.
3   The tendon must run in a straight line in a suitable physiological environment, i.e. unlikely to cause adhesions to form between the tendon and surrounding tissue.

There are certain classical well established muscle and tendon transfer procedures:

1   *For total radial nerve paralysis*
Pronator teres into the extensors carpi radialis.
Flexor carpi ulnaris into extensor digitorum.
Palmeris longus into extensor pollicis longus.

2   *For opponens pollicis paralysis*
Flexor digitorum superficialis to the ring finger passed through a pulley in flexor carpi ulnaris and attached to the postero-radial aspect of the proximal phalanx of the thumb.

3   *For ulnar paralysis*
Extensor carpi radialis brevis prolonged by free tendon grafts which pass volar to the metacarpo-phalangeal joints to be attached to the common extensor tendons on the dorsum of the fingers.

4   *For paralysis of the long finger flexor*
Extensor carpi radialis brevis passed through the interosseous membrane and attached to the deep flexor tendons of the fingers and thumb.

In the hand re-education is usually relatively easy as 'voluntary' control of individual movement is good.

In the legs, movements are largely automatic and muscles normally contract reflexly according to the phase of walking, e.g. in the 'stance' phase the hip and knee extensors and foot plantarflexors contract, in the 'swing' phase the hip and knee flexors and foot dorsiflexors (contract (see Figs. 5.21 and 5.22).

For this reason, it is harder to achieve complete physiological success; nevertheless, certain procedures have proved useful.

5   *For a flexed and adducted hip*
Transfer of the ilio-psoas tendon to the great trochanter.

6   *For a flexed knee knee*
Transfer of the hamstring muscles either to the back of the lower end of the femur or to the patella.

7   *For foot drop* (see common peroneal nerve on page 54).
Transfer of the tibilias posterior through the interosseous membrane to the base of the third metatarsal.

8   *For an inverted foot*
Splitting of the tibialis anterior and transferring it to the outer side of the foot.

Tendon transfers in the foot are often too successful, i.e. they produce the opposite deformities converting an inverted into an everted foot. Each patient must therefore be treated according to his needs.

9   *For pes cavus*
Transferring the peroneus longus and tibialis posterior into the calcaneal tendon.

10   *For claw toes*
Transferring the flexor tendons into the extensor tendons or arthrodese the interphalangeal joints. The metatarso-phalangeal joints must be mobile and not subluxated for these procedures to succeed.

Splints for lesions of the upper limb

Abduction splint

This may be fashioned out of plaster of Paris or be a ready-made splint such as the Littler-Jones abduction splint. The nerve supply to the deltoid muscle which caps the shoulder, is the axillary (circumflex) nerve. This can be damaged in dislocation of the shoulder or in fractures of the surgical neck of the humerus. All fibres of the deltoid muscle abduct the shoulder; the anterior fibres also contribute to flexion; the posterior fibres to extension. The position of abduction at the shoulder ensures that no fibres of the muscle are unduly contracted and none are stretched. Radio (musculo-spinal) nerve splintage.

(i) *The short cock-up splint.* This is used to hold the wrist in an extended position to prevent contractures of the muscles on the anterior surface of the forearm, and to hold the hand and fingers in a functional position.

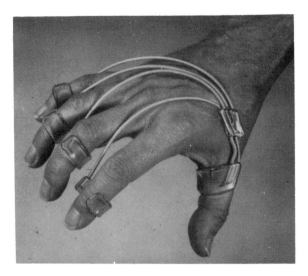

Fig. 3.32. A radial lively splint.

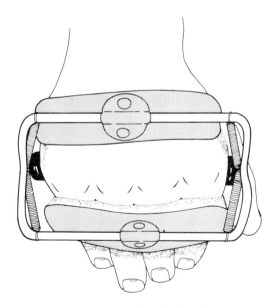

Fig. 3.33. An ulnar lively splint.

(ii) *The radial 'lively' splint* (Fig. 3.32). This consists of a series of springs attached to finger slings. Each finger and the thumb is supported in extension by the springs. Another spring extends the wrist. To flex the fingers, thumb or wrist it is necessary to oppose the pull of the springs. When the flexor muscles relax, the springs pull the wrist, hand and fingers

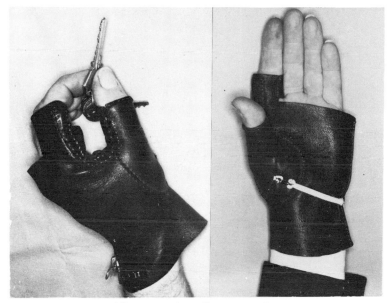

Fig. 3.34. A median nerve splint.

back into the extended position. The patient exercises his functional muscles against the pull of the springs.

Ulnar nerve splint

The ulnar 'lively' splint (Fig. 3.33). This splint opposes the actions of the extensors of the metacarpo-phalangeal joints. If the metacarpal joints are held flexed the long extensor tendons extend the interphalangeal joints.

Median nerve splintage

(See Fig. 3.34). The median nerve enters the palm of the hand under the transverse carpal ligament at the front of the wrist. In the hand it supplies the short muscles which control the thumb, and the skin of the front of the thumb, index fingers, middle finger and the lateral half of the ring finger and corresponding area of the palm. A lesion affecting the median nerve at the wrist causes paralysis of the muscles which flex, oppose and abduct the thumb. A median nerve lesion above the elbow also causes paralysis of the long flexors of the thumb, index and middle finger and of the pronator muscles of the forearm. The hand is then deformed with the fingers and thumb in an extended position with loss of ability to oppose the thumb to the fingers, as in holding a small object. This is described as the 'ape-like' hand because the thumb falls back to lie in the same plane as the fingers.

The median nerve splint is a wrist-band with a loop of material to pull the thumb across the palm of the hand. The thumb can then be opposed to the fingers.

The practical management of patients with peripheral nerve lesions

As with all management of patients the care of the patient with a peripheral nerve lesion requires the cooperation of the many disciplines involved. Thus medicine and surgery, nursing, physiotherapy, occupational therapy, appliance making, medical social work, disablement resettlement officer and other facets of health care are all part of the practical management of the patient. There must be full consultation and organization between the various workers. Peripheral nerve lesions seldom shorten life but they have important economic, recreational and social consequences.

Comprehensive assessment of each patient's problem

Each member of the rehabilitation group must have the opportunity to examine and assess the needs of the patient. This could effectively be broken down to estimation of:
(a)   present condition and problems.
(b)   the requirements to bring the patient to his optimum level of recovery.
(c)   his probable residual paralysis upon discharge from hospital.
(d)   how he may be helped to manage with his permanent disability.
(e)   does he need appliances?
(f)   can he return to his previous form of employment?
(g)   must he be retrained for a new employment?
(h)   if he cannot return to any form of gainful employment how can he be helped financially?
(i)   will he require modification to his home or a change of residence?

An important member of the assessment group is the patient, who must be fully informed and involved. He must know what is being done for him and why. Another person to be considered is the next of kin upon whom the patient will depend for help and support. There is need for conference of all involved in the management of the patient and his problem.

Attitudes to patient management

These will vary according to: (a) the degree of disability, (b) if complete recovery is anticipated, (c) the probability that no recovery will occur.

(a) *The degree of disability:* This is infinitely variable. A peripheral nerve lesion can vary from anaesthesia and temperature changes in a small area of skin to the complete loss of the use of one or more limbs. The patient with a severe disability requires a great deal more encouragement and moral support as well as more vigorous and prolonged efforts to enable him to recover from his disability or to tolerate it if permanent paralysis is present.

(b) *If complete recovery is anticipated:* The approach to management is to ensure that muscles do not waste or atrophy; that joints do not dislocate or become stiff, deformed and unusable; that skin is whole and healthy and without ulcers or scars; that the patient has as full a range of locomotion as existed prior to the lesion when full recovery occurs.

(c) *The probability that no recovery will occur:* In this situation the patient must be mentally orientated and trained to live the remainder of his life with a problem which can vary from slight to severe. This may be:

(a) retraining to manage his occupation when his salient limb is weak,

(b) coping within the regime dictated by his crutches, calipers or splints,

(c) management of all life including occupation, from a wheelchair,

(d) accepting a life to be spent mainly within the confines of his own home.

Local management of the affected part

When skin is deprived of a sensory nerve supply the patient is unaware of pain or sensation. Thus he has no knowledge of pressure, constriction, burning or any other injury. He is unaware that anything is wrong. He must, therefore, learn to protect the anaesthetic and paralysed limb.

The anaesthetic skin must be kept clean, dry and free from local compressions, such as crumbs in creases of skin, buttons and metal tags on clothing, stones in shoes or body pressure on it when lying or sitting. Such simply trauma as may be caused by a bad darn or a tight supporting strap or band on clothing can be serious.

The denervated area must also be protected from extremes of heat or cold. Hot-water bottles, hot plates, lit cigarettes, hot-water taps, radiators, and stoves are all hazards; in cold weather the hand or foot, if involved, must be covered by a loosely fitting glove or sock. Strong chemicals or washing detergents may also be a danger.

Manicure of the hands or pedicure of the feet should only be performed, on the paralysed side, by an expert. Trimming of corns and callosities must only by done by a trained chiropodist.

Involvement of the autonomic nervous supply reduces the efficiency of the venous return from the limb. Thus engorgement of the blood vessels with oedema and swelling will occur if the limb is allowed to hang down for a long time. Another danger is that a joint which is deprived of its supporting cuff of muscles may dislocate or a joint deprived of sensory innervation may disintegrate—the so-called Charcot or neuropathic joint. For paralysis of the leg, the patient should sit with the affected limb raised so that the foot is level with the pelvis. When the arm or hand is paralysed the upper limb should rest on a table when the patient sits, so that the hand is level with the shoulder. Pillows or supports in the bed for the affected limb may also be necessary.

Physical therapy will include:

1   The prevention of contraction of the capsules of the joints at sites where no patient instigated movement can occur. If, when recovery of muscles occurs, the joints are immovable treatment will be either prolonged or fail. Passive exercises are used for this.

2   Re-education of paralysed muscles, as recovery from the palsy occurs, by the use of active exercises.

3   Electrical stimulation of muscles, during paralysis, to prevent loss of muscle bulk and minimize wasting.

4   Ordering, fitting and supervision of 'lively' splintage to ensure that this is serving the purpose for which it is supplied.

5   Estimation and recording, frequently, the amount of recovery occurring in an individual muscle.

6   Teaching and supervising new methods of locomotion when walking is impaired because of leg paralysis.

Occupation therapy will include:

1   Assessment of the problems of the patient and the rate and amount of recovery anticipated.

2   The means of collaborating with the physiotherapy staff to avoid contractures and stiffness in the affected joints.

3   The best methods of re-educating muscles undergoing recovery.

4   Treatment to prevent wasting and disuse atrophy of the paralysed muscles.

5   Teaching methods of vital activity, e.g. dressing and washing, shaving and feeding with residual paralysis affecting upper or lower limbs.

6   Demonstrating and arranging to supply equipment to help the patient manage his daily living with independence.

7   Cooperating with the disablement resettlement officer in preparing the patient for a return to employment.

Causalgia

The word causalgia is frequently applied in a rather loose sense to any painful clinical syndrome of the limbs following an injury either to a peripheral nerve, a plexus or even to the cauda equina and spinal cord. This loose use of the term is undesirable as causalgia embraces a very specific clinical entity. Some pain, or at least unpleasant sensations are the normal accompaniment of recovery or partial nerve lesions. Similarly, irritation of the nerve root will give rise to pain as is seen classically in sciatica and brachial neuritis due to disc lesions or other causes. Equally, disease processes such as tumours of secondary deposits in the spine will give rise to pain, but none of these should be properly termed causalgia.

Basically, the causalgic syndrome is when a patient suffers from severe spontaneous, burning pain associated with a peripheral nerve lesion which is usually incomplete. In particular causalgic phenomena are associated with partial damage to the median or medial popliteal nerves, usually in the proximal part of the limb. Not only is the pain of a peculiarly intense and burning character and is present spontaneously, but certain factors aggravate the pain, particularly heat, emotion, worry, sexual excitement, noise, fear, in fact the pain is aggravated by any external or internal stimulus which would normally cause stimulation of the sympathetic nervous system. Similarly, the pain is relieved by certain measures which damp down sympathetic activity. The individual may sit in a dark quiet corner with his hand wrapped in a flannel wrung out in ice-cold water, and refuse to participate in social contact. He may be terrified of anything that might upset him; in particular, noise, excitement or fear. Even the sight of somebody else walking down the ward on crutches will aggravate his pain because he will be anxious less they should slip and fall over. These features are so pronounced that sometimes the patient is accused of being psychiatrically disturbed.

The clinical signs are usually those of a partial lesion associated with a proximal site of wounding and as already stated, the median and the medial popliteal nerves are the most frequent nerves to be affected. There will be hyperhydrosis (excessive sweating) in the region of distribution of the nerve; small blisters will often form on the skin and the colour of the affected part is plum-coloured. There will also be evidence of trophic disturbances, e.g. the hand or foot will be swollen at the joints which are stiff but the digital pulses will atrophy. The radiograph shows periarticular osteoporosis.

It is generally considered that the true causalgic syndrome is due to a breakdown of insulation between the autonomic fibres and the afferent pain transmitting fibres. The theory is that the autonomic fibres transmitting electrical impulses from the centre to the periphery which control blood vessels, pilomotor activity, sweating and so on, stimulate the afferent, pain-conducting fibres directly. Therefore any stimulus, physical or emotional, which would normally cause increased activity or the sympathetic nervous system will automatically stimulate pain fibres.

The trophic phenomena, that is the plum-coloured congested hand, the excessive sweating, blistering and so on, are attributed to disturbance of the axon reflex. The fact that the overwhelming majority of patients with true causalgia are cured of their causalgic syndrome by efficient sympathectomy suggests that this theory is fundamentally correct, at best it fits in with all the observed clinical data. Of course, following a successful sympathectomy for causalgia the patient may still have some residual tenderness, some dysaesthesia such as is associated with any partial or recovering nerve lesion. In addition, during the period of causalgia there will have been considerable trophic changes in muscles, bones and joints, leading to patchy osteoporosis particularly adjacent to the joints. This appearance is in some way analogous to what is seen in rheumatoid arthritis. The joints will be stiff and the capsules will have lost their normal elasticity and be fibrotic. In the process of mobilizing these joints to restore function, the patient will probably experience some pain but it will be different in nature from the severe and overwhelming pain of causalgia.

Pain following division of a major peripheral nerve and particularly pain following an amputation has next to be considered; It is, of course, normal after an amputation for the patient to experience what is known as the phantom limb phenomenon. He or she, feels as if their limb were still present. They often feel even that the amputated digits are moving. They refer the position of their absent limb in space to rather nearer the body axis than it was before the amputation. These phantom limbs can be unpleasant and misleading and often associated with an unpleasant tingling. They also present the danger that the patient may forget that his leg has been amputated and may attempt to stand or walk on the non-existent foot, thus falling over and perhaps badly damaging the healing amputation stump. Most patients of stable temperament accept the presence of these phantoms if it is explained to them and gradually the phantom sensations become weaker and almost fade away and do not seriously disturb the patient.

Occasionally, however, the phantom limb is associated with severe pain. The exact reason for this is uncertain, but it does seem that the incidence of painful phantoms is increased if the damage to the limb is sustained under peculiarly emotional circumstances, if the patient has an unstable temperament, if there is excessive resentment or if there are important medico-legal considerations. All these factors appear to increase the insidence of painful phantoms, but there is a great deal that is inexplicable.

For instance, sometimes one sees patients who have managed quite well for a number of years and suddenly something happens to produce painful phantoms of the amputated limb. In certain circumstances, local factors, for example, a large terminal neuroma adherent to skin or bone or subjected to gross trauma, may be contributory factors. Under other circumstances, changes in the blood supply to the nerve, for example or ischaemia with increasing age may also appear to be responsible. In general, attention to the major nerves at the time of the primary amputation ensuring that they are clean-cut and that they are allowed to retract in among muscle and are not adherent to bone or skin appear to diminish the risk of painful phantoms developing. Nevertheless, when one has said all this, one is conscious of the fact that we do not fully understand this phenomenon and that a vast number of treatments, for example, division or crushing the nerve at a higher level, injecting it with local anaesthetic, performing sympathectomies, re-amputation or even division of sensory nerve roots, cordotomy and leucotomies may all fail completely to relieve the symptoms.

The most popular theory is that in some vaguely understood way there is competition in the ascending tracts of the spinal cord between sensory impulses of various kinds and if the tracts carrying impulses which produce the sensations of pain are uninhibited, the patient will experience pain. If on the other hand, the various tracts are fully occupied transmitting other impulses, the pain component in the total sensory image will be much less. A patient experiences pain when noxious or unpleasant stimulae are in the majority and there is an absence of balancing stimulae. If there has been a predominance of painful impulses over a certain period, then the central nervous system appears to be conditioned and even if the original peripheral cause of the painful stimulus is eliminated, impulses travelling up the ascending tract of the spinal cord are still predominantly of a type which produce painful sensations in the sensorium. Admittedly this theory is a very vague one and is more in the nature of a speculation than based on anatomical and physiological evidence, yet it would appear that our final subjective interpretation of the activities of sensory neurones at all levels, is a complex phenomenon in which a large number of different type of impulses participate and a balance between thalamo-cortical, spino-thalamic, spino-cortical impulses all must take place. There is perhaps, an analogy here to pain following an injury to the spinal cord. It is well recognized that absence of interest in life, absence of occupation and failure of rehabilitation increase the incidence of pain after spinal cord injuries. There are considerable similarities between post-amputation painful stumps and post-paraplegic painful spines.

PARALYSIS IN LEPROSY

Leprosy has largely disappeared in most industrialized countries, and effective treatment can render an affected individual non-infectious within 6–8 weeks, so that it is anticipated that ultimately the number of lepers will diminish drastically. Nevertheless, at the moment there are some millions of affected individuals, and in many of these the disease affects one or more peripheral nerves. It is not known for certain how the lepra bacilli reach the peripheral nerves. Some authorities believe that the spread is via the lymphatic system, others that it is a centripetal spread from tubercoloid skin patches. The reaction in an individual's nerves depends on a number of complex factors, including the virulence and quantity of the infecting agent and the individual's response.

The first evidence of infection by 'Hanson's bacillus' is often the individual's awareness of one or more areas of anaesthetic skin—the so-called tuberculoid reaction. Presumably, the nerve endings are already affected at this stage. Examination may reveal thickening of one of the accessibale superficial nerves such as the posterior auricular. At this stage, medicinal treatment with, for example, dapsone, will halt the progress of the infection and render the individual non-infective. A number of clinical syndromes can be recognized.

Acute pain

However occasionally, there is acute hypersensitivity reaction to treatment when one or more peripheral nerves become acutely swollen, and the patient experiences severe pain in the distribution of the nerve. Fortunately, this acute reaction usually subsides with treatment with steroids—formerly it was advised that a longitudinal incision should be made in the swollen nerve, but this is rarely indicated nowadays.

Chronic pain

Sometimes the patient complains of intolerable long continued pain in the distribution of a nerve which is the site of extensive intraneural fibrosis. This is a difficult and intractable condition for which a number of procedures—both external and internal neurolysis—have been advocated, but the evidence for their effectiveness is as yet somewhat dubious.

Paralysis

It is a peculiarity of leprosy that only superficial portions of peripheral nerves are involved. Thus, the ulnar nerve is commonly affected at the elbow; the media nerve at the wrist, the common peroneal nerve where it winds round the neck of the fibula, the posteror tibial nerve at the ankle and the facial nerve are the most important nerves to be affected. Occasionally, the musculo-spiral nerve is involved at the elbow.

Although some surgeons believe that decompression can lead to recovery of motor function, the evidence for this is not at the moment universally accepted. Nevertheless, procedures such as dividing the transverse carpal ligament or the fascia between the two heads of the flexor carpi ulnaris are very minor procedures and at least do no harm, so it is not unreasonable to consider such operations when the paralysis is of recent onset. The operation must, of course, be accompanied by specific chemotherapy.

For established paralysis, where there is no hope of muscular recovery, a number of well established procedures are available.

Foot drop

For the foot drop due to common peroneal nerve palsy, transplanting the tibialis posterior through the interosseous membrane to the dorsum of the foot is a well-established and highly-successful manoeuvre. Preferably, the tendon should then be split in two and one half attached to the medial, the other half to the lateral border of the foot. This 'stirrup' arrangement ensures that the foot becomes plantigrade, and does not assume either an inverted or everted position. Retraining of the tibialis muscle to perform its new function is usually easy, but it helps if the physiotherapist has been able to spend some time with the patient before operation, and has taught him to perform static isometric contractions of the tibialis posterior, while trying to 'image' dorsiflexion and eversion of the foot.

Intrinsic paralysis

A large number of different procedures have been devised for the typical claw hand of ulnar paralysis. Some surgeons claim that it is enough to prevent hyperextension of the metacarpo-phalangeal joints by a tenodesis, but most surgeons find that Paul Brand's procedure of using free tendon grafts to connect the extensor carpi radialis tendon to the extensor tendons in the fingers is the most effective. The tendon grafts are routed between the metacarpal bones from posterior to anterior, and then run along the course of the lumbrical tendons to be attached to the extensor tendon expansion at the level of the proximal phalanx. Naturally, it is important before operation to ensure that there are no fixed-joint deformities and that the donor muscle (extensor carpi radialis brevis) is acting sufficiently strongly. After operation, the hand must be splinted in the 'intrinsic-plus' position for three weeks. Retraining of the leprosy hand is then usually relatively easy — possibly due to diminished pain sensitivity, though in the presence of anaesthesia, great care must be taken not to cause injury to the skin or joints.

Median nerve paralysis

The median nerve in leprosy is involved at the wrist, so that the forearm muscles are usually acting normally. The question of which muscles are available to provide motor power to restore the power of opposition will obviously depend on the degree of ulnar nerve involvement.

If both flexor tendons to the ring finger are active, the superficial flexor tendon to the ring finger can be used. A loop is formed out of part of the flexor carpi ulnaris, and the tendon passed through this loop, then across the palm to be inserted on the radial aspect of the thumb metacarpophalangeal joint. If this tendon is not available, the corresponding tendon of the middle finger may be used or, less successfully, one of the finger extensor tendons.

Facial paralysis

In addition to the cosmetic blemish, inability to close the eye may lead to corneal ulceration. Fortunately, an excellent procedure exists, namely to use the temporalis muscle and its fascia and route strips of the fascia round the eyes. Similarly, the muscle can be used to elevate the corner of the mouth. Re-education is surprisingly easy and effective.

Anaesthesia

This is undoubtedly the unsolved outstanding problem of leprosy. Serious damage to an anaesthetic hand can be avoided by constant vigilance on the patient's part, but if he is careless he may gradually lose all his fingers. Obviously, anaesthesia greatly reduces the functioned capacity of the hand-skilled movements, which are dependent on adequate 'feed back' from the periphery.

In the case of the foot anaesthesia of the sole due to posterior tibial involvement, this is a very serious problem. Again, constant vigilance by the patient is essential. In addition, the provision of suitable footwear is a great help. Essentially, there should be a rigid under sole with a rocker under the metatarsal heads, but a soft inner sole moulded to the foot's shape (often cavus due to intrinsic muscle paralysis), a suitable shoe is shown in Figure 3.35.

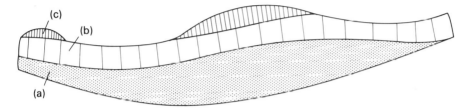

Fig. 3.35. Simple sandal for patients with anaesthetic feet. (a) Firm rocker-shaped sole, e.g. wood and vulcanized rubber. (b) Soft moulded insole, e.g. micropore rubber. (c) Special build up of felt in instep and under toes.

If an anaesthetic foot is neglected, intractable ulceration, chronic infection, osteomyelitis and bone destruction may lead to amputation. Even without this, neuropathic disintegration of joints may necessitate the use of supporting irons.

4 : Affections of Skeletal Muscles and Tendons

Relevant anatomy and physiology

The skeletal muscles have the following functions:

1   To support the trunk an any chosen position; thus standing or sitting requires muscles to hold the body in a stable posture.

2   To stabilize the synovial joints of the limbs so that the limbs may be placed and held in the position in which they are required.

3   To move the synovial joints, and thus the body. Movements such as walking, running and jumping are caused by muscles.

4   To contract and apply precise controlled and varying amounts of pressure. Thus small 'feint' movements or powerful thrusts or pressures are equally required from any given muscle.

5   To prevent stasis in the tissues; the muscles have 'tone' they contribute to the firm 'feel' of the tissues and cause movement when they are under pressure; they apply intermittent pressure to the blood vessels and thus help venous return.

6   To contribute to the activities within the abdominal cavity by varying the pressures as they compress the contents.

7   To cause respiration by varying the volume of the thoracic cavity as the walls of the chest are moved by muscle tissue.

8   To assist communication with others by varying facial expressions.

This list of functions may be developed *ad infinitum* as the muscles contribute to most of the functions of the body.

SKELETAL MUSCLES AND POSTURE

The bony skeleton has the best shape and size for the functions it is required to perform. The length and weight of the individual bones, their shape and their balance all form part of a pattern. This pattern requires minimal muscle power to enable the skeleton to stay upright in standing, to cause motion in walking, running and jumping, to vary the pressures in the thorax and to permit bending and stretching in many directions. The muscles attached to the skeleton both cause movement at the joints and also hold the joints still when needed.

A major factor in reducing the quantity of muscular effort needed to hold or move the skeleton is the centring of the mass of the skeleton and its attached tissues over the base (see Fig. 4.1). Thus, when posture is good, the centre of gravity, which is normally in front of the lumbar curve, is accurately placed over the centre of the feet when standing. To keep the skeleton upright and the centre of gravity over the feet a minimal amount of muscle effort, applied intermittently to pull the body in the required direction is all that is needed.

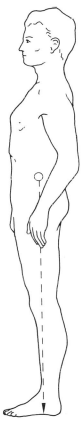

Fig. 4.1. When posture is normal the centre of gravity (represented by the circle on the abdomen of this figure) is centred over the base. If a plumb-line is dropped from the centre of gravity (were this possible) it would end at a point exactly between the feet. Minimum muscular effort is needed to support this posture.

When the body is distorted by deformity, the centre of gravity is usually moved away from its correct position to one side or even in extreme examples to the edge of the base almost outside of the area of the base. Thus an attempt to bring the centre of gravity to a more stable position requires much more muscular effort, and standing, walking or even sitting is a far more exhausting process. It follows that patients who have severe deformities, affecting the shape of the skeleton, will become exhausted more quickly than when there is no deformity and the body is upright over its base. To add to the patient's problems his thorax is also often inadequate in volume because of the misshapen skeleton and the oxygen intake will not satisfy the needs of the muscles and tissues; thus they do not function efficiently and weakness and lethargy will result.

Balance

All body function and posture requires a coordinated balance of muscular activites. One group of muscles is opposed to another and thus when they pull with equal force a joint is held in a stable, fixed, position; when one group pulls with more strength than the other a movement is caused and the group of muscles not causing the movement relax to permit it to happen but they contract again at the end of the movement so as to restore stability. In this way the movements of the joints of the trunk, neck and limbs are controlled and the movements are smooth, accurate and precise provided the nervous system is functioning normally.

Imbalance

The opposite of controlled movement is incoordinating ataxia or jerkiness. This happens when the balance of the muscles is disordered either when the central nervous system is abnormal, or a peripheral nerve lesion (Chapter 3) exists, when there is imbalance the two opposing groups of muscles are not coordinated either because one group is pulling too fiercely or that the other is not opposing strongly enough, or is paralysed or diseased. There will then exist:
(a)   disordered movements such as spasticity, jerkiness, tremor, athetosis, ataxia, clonus or tics.
(b)   deformity, such as flexion extension contractures, when the shape of the limb is grossly distorted.

Diseases of muscle

Diseases of muscle may be either intrinsic or extrinsic.

Extrinsic causes

Extrinsic causes can be divided into neurogenic and vascular. In neurogenic diseases of muscle there is an affection of either an anterior horn cell of the spinal cord, or of a motor nerve; this leads to paralysis, wasting and finally degeneration of the muscle fibres, with loss of electrical excitability so that the normal brisk response to an interrupted electric current (faradic current) is lost and the muscle will only respond sluggishly, either at the start or at the end of a continuous (galvanic) stimulation (Fig. 4.2).

Vascular disorders of muscle are usually due to impairment of the arterial blood supply; this leads to death of the muscle cells, loss of contractility, replacement by scar tissue, fibrosis and contracture (Volkmann's

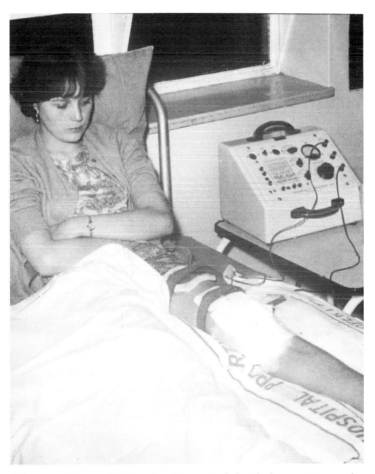

Fig. 4.2. The application of an interrupted electrical current to muscle.

ischaemic contracture). Such disorders usually occur in association with fractures, e.g. supracondylar fractures of the elbow in children, either as a sequel to spasm of the artery or to contusion of the wall of the artery and thrombosis with obliteration of the lumen (see Fig. 8.9b).

Similarly, the blood supply may be cut off by venous obstruction with back pressure on the capillaries and ultimately cessation of the circulation. Minor degrees of muscle ischaemia are probably very common in association with fractures, particularly fractures of the tibia, and on occasions fractures of the femur may be associated with major damage to the femoral artery and ischaemia of the below-knee muscles which may lead to deformities of the foot, such as an equinus deformity due to contracture of the calf muscle.

Intrinsic disease in muscle

A number of conditions loosely linked together under the title of 'myopathies' have been described. In general these occur in early childhood, e.g. about the age of five years, and become progressively worse during the growing period, ultimately leading to widespread weakness. A number of different clinical types have been described. The commonest is the so-called pseudohypertrophic type which particularly affects the calf, quadriceps and trunk muscles so that the patient has difficulty in standing and getting up from the lying position. He tends to have a characteristic posture and a lurching, waddling gait, with an exaggerated lordosis (Fig. 4.3). The condition is more common in boys and is usually caused by a sex-linked dominant gene.

Muscle wasting and weakness may occur in a wide variety of other conditions—e.g. in the presence of malignant disease and particularly in carcinoma of the bronchus; in association with diabetes, and with various forms of chronic arthritis; various endocrine disorders—e.g. thyroid and adrenal disorders, and in association with a number of rare disorders of carbohydrate metabolism.

The whole subject of primary muscle disease is a difficult and complex one and in every case of marked muscle wasting it is important to institute a thorough investigation of the causes which may include electrical tests, electromyography and muscle biopsy. Often the primary disease cannot be treated, but orthopaedic treatment—physiotherapy, preventing and correcting deformities, supporting apparatus, and stabilizing operations, may help the patient to remain mobile.

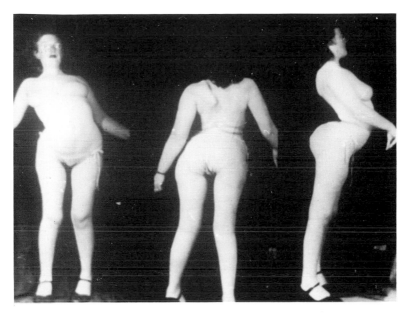

Fig. 4.3.   The exaggerated lordosis of muscular dystrophy.

Nerves and muscles

The efficient function of muscles depends upon communication with the spinal cord and the brain. In the transmission of instructions from the brain to the muscles, efferent or motor nerves carry the impulses; thus every muscle, no matter how small, must be supplied with a motor nerve branch. For coordinated activity of the whole body, the brain and spinal cord must be fully informed of every change in position in a muscle; afferent or sensory nerves constantly carry impulses (electrical messages) back to the central nervous system; every muscle must therefore also have afferent, sensory nerve fibres communicating from the muscle to the spinal cord and brain. Any interruption in either the motor or sensory nerve supply of a muscle results in serious impairment of the function of the muscle. There must be communication for there to be proper control.

Muscle denervation

There are a number of syndromes connected with diseases of muscle. In the first place, of course, if there is untreated spasticity of a muscle it may lead to contracture. Contrarywise if there is a lower motor neurone lesion of muscle, that is, a denervation syndrome (Fig. 4.4) this may lead to either permanent lengthening of the muscle or occasionally to fibrosis and shortening.

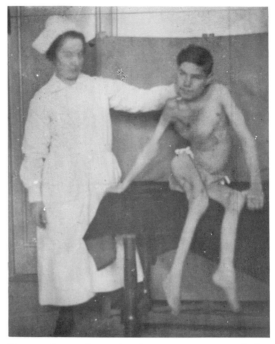

Fig. 4.4.   Denervation syndrome in a lower motor neurone lesion of muscle.

Blood vessels, blood and muscles

All the tissues of the body must have an adequate supply of circulating blood. The amount required by muscles is larger than that of many tissues; there is a direct relationship between the work performed and the quantity of blood needed by muscular tissue. When work is performed by a muscle there must be a corresponding supply of nutrient material such as glucose and oxygen. The greater the amount of work, the more nutrition and oxygen carrying blood the muscle will require. Every muscle has arteries, carrying oxygenated blood into the tissues, and veins carrying de-oxygenated blood away from the tissues.

Impairment or complete cessation of the blood supply to any tissue or organ is a serious matter; the function of the tissue will be reduced or the tissue will die.

Muscle ischaemia

The disorder of muscle which is unfortunately only too common is fibrosis secondary to ischaemia. This may be either due to an injury leading to obliteration of blood supply to the muscle. This is very common in certain injuries around the elbow, particularly supracondylar fractures, or it may occur secondary to injection of antibiotics into the muscle. It seems that children under five years of age are specially susceptible to this.

Collagen tissue

The different organs of the body are linked together by connective tissue. Connective tissue also plays an important part in maintaining the shape of individual organs and muscles.

Collagen is a complex protein which is found in the body in the white fibres of connective tissue. It forms about one third of muscle and about one third of bone. In butchers' meat and bone the collagen is converted to gelatine when boiled.

In muscle, white fibrous tissue is an important supporting structure which is essential for the conversion of the contractility of the muscle cells into mechanical work as it creates a structure against which the muscle cells can pull and push.

Tendons are mainly collagen. Collagen is also found in the capsules of joints which are composed mainly of fibrous tissue.

Collagen disorders

There is a group of muscle disorders in which there is deficiency of the collagen tissue as seen in conditions like the Marfan syndrome or the Ehlers-Danlos syndrome. Apart from these classical syndromes there are a number of children who have hypermobile joints (Fig. 4.5) and poorly developed, floppy muscles—not quite a flaccid paralysis but very nearly. The primary disorder appears to be in the collagen tissue, and of course, it is on the integrity of the collagen tissue that the muscle fibres depend in order to transmit their contractions into mechanical work.

The neuromuscular junction

Where a nerve enters muscle tissue the nerve impulse is transferred from the nerve tissue to the muscle tissue. This causes the muscle to respond to the nerve impulse, by contracting. At this neuromuscular junction there

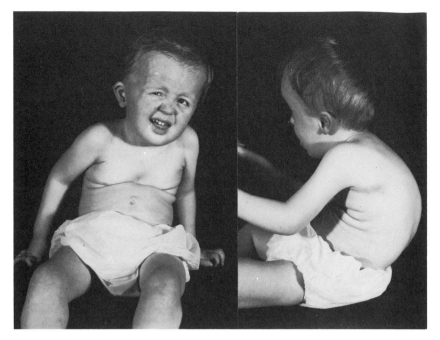

Fig. 4.5. A child with hypermobile joints.

is the release of a chemical called acetylcholine which is stored in small vesicles in the enlarged nerve ending. For the muscle to contract it is essential that acetylcholine passes across a gap between membranes at the junction of the nerve and the muscle tissue.

Acetylcholine increases the rate at which potassium and sodium ions pass across membranes and thus cause conduction across a synapse. Each time a nerve impulse arrives it causes the release of acetylcholine which results in a muscle contraction.

Myasthenia gravis

Myasthenia gravis is a condition in which there is a failure of transmission of the nervous impulse from the nerve to the muscle, and this disease is characterized by progressive weakness, the muscles quickly becoming tired. It does appear that there is a basic deficiency in the formation and transference of acetylcholine at the nerve endings which are responsible for transmission of the nervous impulse from the nerve to the muscle. Considerable success in treatment has been obtained by giving substitution chemotherapy, such as physostigmine, to the patient.

Metabolic disorders of muscles

There are a group of what one may call 'metabolic disorders of muscle' in which there is widespread weakness and myopathy. They are often associated with conditions like diabetes or evidence of malignant disease elsewhere in the body. It is not fully understood how these metabolic effects produce this meakness but when one sees otherwise inexplicable weakness and wasting of muscles one must think of one or other of these constitutional diseases.

POLYMYOSITIS

This is a relatively rare condition sometimes known as polymyositis or dermatomyositis in which there is widespread weakness of the muscles often associated with patches of thickening and discoloration of the skin. This is a disease of unknown aetiology; it is possible that there is some connection with the rheumatic diseases though it does not respond to cortisone: it appears to respond to immuno-suppressive drugs.

MYOSITIS OSSIFICANS

The long bones of the body ossify in cartilage. This ossification is caused by the activity of specialized bone cells which convert soft cartilaginous tissue into solid bone. In the process of growth in length of a long bone, first the cartilage cells divide. The cartilage is then invaded by osteoblasts so that solidification occurs at the growth cartilages at the bone ends. To increase the diameter of long bones, new bone is laid down in layers like the growth rings of a tree, underneath the periosteum, the membrane surrounding the long bones. This also occurs in the repair of bone after fracture. Simultaneously bone on the inner aspect of the cortex is absorbed so that the medullary cavity enlarges with growth.

There is obscure disease of muscles in which the muscles are gradually replaced by bone, sometimes known as myositis ossificans universalis (Fig. 4.6). Again this disease is of unknown aetiology and there is no specific treatment.

This condition occurs in two forms: a localized form may occur following injury—in particular the brachialis muscle in front of the elbow and the quadriceps muscle in front of the thigh are the two commonest sites, but minor degrees may occur in other situations. It is believed that osteogenic cells grow into a haematoma and form bone there.

Basically the treatment is to rest the condition in the acute phase and, as the acute phase settles down, graduated exercises are introduced. Massage and forced movements only aggravate the condition.

Chapter 4

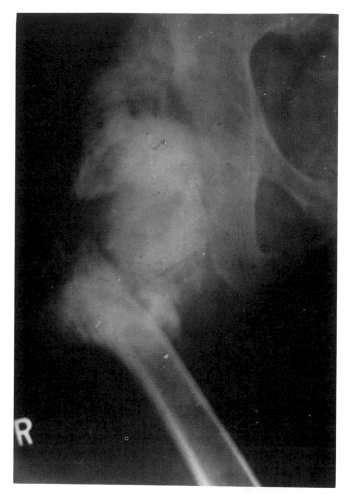

Fig. 4.6. A radiograph to show myositis ossificans.

The generalized form of myositis ossificans is extremely rare; the cause is unknown but it is a progressive condition in which the skeletal muscles are gradually replaced by bone causing progressive stiffness, deformity, and ultimately complete immobility usually leading to death from respiratory infection. No effective treatment is known.

CONGENITAL ABSENCE OF MUSCLES

Certain muscles may be congenitally absent. The commonest example is the pectoralis major. Usually there is realtively little functional disability and the main problem is the cosmetic blemish. Progressive fibrosis and shortening of muscle may occur as a sequel to multiple injections (e.g. of antibiotics in infancy). This results in progressive diminution of the range of movement—e.g. if the quadriceps is affected, the range of flexion is decreased. To correct lengthen the tendon of the affected muscle or to separate the affected part from the normal part of the muscle.

ARTHROGRYPOSIS

This is an uncommon congenital condition in which the child is born with multiple deformities, widespread replacement of muscle tissue by fibrous tissue, and a peculiar abnormality of the subcutaneous tissue and fascia so that the normal flexion creases in the skin are absent and the child's limbs have a curious smooth 'seal-like' appearance. It is common for such children to have club feet, flexed knees, dislocated hips; in some minor cases the condition occurs affecting only a few muscles. Basically the treatment is to correct deformities by lengthening contracted muscles and tendons and also joint capsules; if necessary, corrective osteotomies of of bone are performed. There may be associated congenital anomalies of the skeleton.

THE MUSCULAR DYSTROPHIES (Fig. 4.7)

There are a number of types of these but the commonest and most serious is the so-called pseudohypertrophic form which usually manifests itself about the age of four or five. It occurs commonly in boys, is inherited as a dominant sex-linked disorder and leads to increasing paralysis and weakness usually ending in death before the age of twenty. The calf muscles, the gluteal muscles and the trunk muscles are first affected leading to progressive waddling gait and inability to get up from the sitting or lying position. Another not uncommon type of muscle dystrophy is the so-called facio-scapulo-humeral muscle dystrophy which comes on at a later age and does not progress so rapidly. Both these conditions may be associated with weakness of the cardiac muscle which is another cause of death. It is not sex linked and the relevant gene is usually recessive.

Occasionally in facio-scapulo-humeral dystrophy where the patient has difficulty in using their arms, he can he helped by surgical operations to fix the scapula to the rib cage.

Another type is the Charcot-Marie-Tooth muscle dystrophy which primarily affects the dorsiflexor and evertor muscles of the leg and pro-

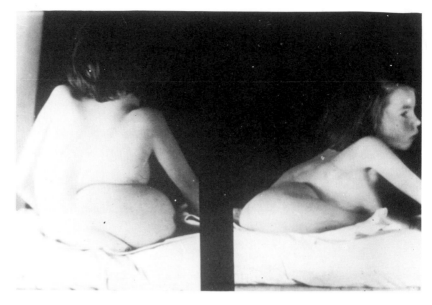

Fig. 4.7. A patient with muscular dystrophy.

duces an equino-caro-cavus deformity of the feet. This also usually has an hereditary basis, but is not sex linked. The small muscles of the hand may be affected.

Lastly, in late adult life there is a relatively benign type of muscle dystrophy: this also seems to be inherited. It leads to progressive weakness especially of the neck muscles. There is no known specific treatment but supporting orthopaedic measures can help.

The management of patients with pseudohypertrophic muscular dystrophy

The management of the patients with this condition requires management of the family also. Often there is a history of the condition in previous generations of the mother's family and they are fully aware of the prognosis. It may be that several or all of the children of the current generation are affected.

The parents will notice that the child is later than others of similar age in standing and walking and their attention is drawn to the condition by the peculiar waddling gait, the tendency to fall over and severe difficulty in getting up from a lying position. To do this the child develops a trick pattern to compensate for the weakness of the extensors of the hip and the contractures of the flexors of the hip. This consists of (a) rolling over on to the anterior surface of the body, (b) flexing the hips to push the buttocks from the ground, (c) struggling on to the feet in a crouched posture and (d) using the hands and arms to 'climb up' his own skeleton and eventually he stands upright with a lordotic posture (Fig. 4.8).

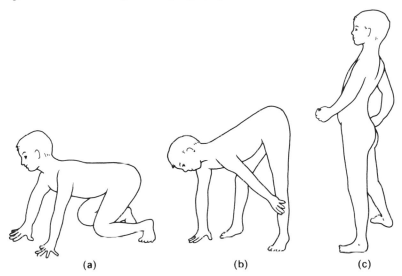

(a)   (b)   (c)

Fig. 4.8.   A muscular dystrophy patient climbing up his own limbs to stand up.

The muscles contain little or no contractile tissue and thus, they are weak and ineffectual. This progresses until the patient becomes completely confined to a wheelchair or bed.

The management of such young people requires much physical effort on the part of the attendants as the patient must be lifted from chair to bed or chair to toilet when the condition has progressed to an advanced stage. If there is more than one patient in the family the hard work required to maintain the patient is prolonged and unremitting.

The family therefore must have relief. Special schools, social clubs and institutions exist for the care of these patients. If the muscular dystrophy child can board at a school for most of the week and return to parent care (when possible) at weekends or holidays a reasonable existence is possible for both the parents and the patients. In the home full use of hoists, cranes and other mechanicl devices and modifications to the house to assist lifting and wheelchair movement are essential. Equipment such as washing machines and related labour-saving devices are necessary in the home where progressively deteriorating invalids are to be managed. Heavy financial support from the social security or other state benefits are necessary to relieve the tremendous strain on the budget which the management of such patients can cause.

The physiotherapist and occupational therapist have a major role in assisting the family and patients. The physiotherapist assists by retarding the development of fixed contractures and by keeping the muscles as active as their limited contractibility will allow.

Occupational therapy and muscular dystrophy

The occupational therapist assists by helping the patient and family to establish as reasonable a pattern of living as possible and providing an occupation to give an outlet for the mental and physical abilities of the patient. As the muscular range will decrease there must be limitation of the physical effort, required to perform a task related to the deteriorating muscle power.

As deterioration in muscular dystrophy is gradual and extending over many years there may be little, at first, for the occupational therapist to do to help the patient; perhaps an introduction to establish an interest in hobbies which the patient can continue to practice when his range of activities is severely restricted. It is when the patient has problems in occupational activity or in his normal daily living routine that he will require more vigorous help.

Possibly the most serious problem to be handled is the depression associated with an increasing awareness by the patient of his dependence upon his family for the maintenance of personal standards. This deterioration in morale can have an adverse effect on other members of the family.

The main approach to management is to assist the patient to keep his independence for as long as possible. Careful frequent assessment by the rehabilitation unit is necessary however to ensure that the patient is not exhausting himself in his efforts to avoid the help of others.

5 : Acute Lesions of the Spinal Cord

Definitions

Paraplegia is the condition which exists when some or all of the nerve tracts or pathways in the spinal cord have been interrupted or severed below the level of thoracic segment number 2 or 3, or lower, and as a result there is paralysis of both lower extremities.

Tetraplegia exists when some or all of the pathways or nerve tracts of the spinal cord have been interrupted or severed at the level of thoracic segment number 2 or higher. In this instance the paralysis affects all of the limbs. The higher the lesion the greater the paralysis.

Relevant applied anatomy and physiology

The spinal cord passes down the neural canal of the vertebral column to the level of the first and second lumbar vertebrae. Below where this has terminated nerves forming the cauda equina continue to the lowest point of the neural canal.

The brain and spinal cord, with their coverings, constitute the main control centres of the body. They are composed of nervous tissue which is sensitive, soft and vulnerable to damage. Therefore, they must be protected in a special bony and membranous covering.

The bony protection is provided by a cavity situated inside the skull and vertebral column which is entirely surrounded by hard bone which is sufficient protection from the normal stresses and trauma which will be applied to the body in everyday activites. Even a hard blow to the head or back will not usually affect the enclosed nervous tissue. Extreme force will, however, breach this defence.

The spinal cord is the trunk of nerve tissue which provides communication between the brain and the remainder of the body. It contains the pathways by which nerve impulses are conveyed from brain to muscles, blood vessels, viscera and skin; from muscles, tendons and joints to the brain in the reverse direction. Interruption of these pathways means that there is no communication between the structure at each end of each pathway.

As the peripheral pathways (peripheral nerves) leave the spinal cord at the first convenient point adjacent to the part they serve they will only be involved in a lesion of the cord if that lesion occurs above the point where the relevant spinal nerve leaves the spinal cord. It follows, therefore, that the lower down the lesion in the cord, the less the disability which results, and the higher the lesion, the greater the disability will be. If the lesion is above the fourth cervical level the patient usually dies immediately. Thus, a patient with a sacral lesion will be less disabled than one with a lumbar lesion; a patient with a lumbar lesion will be less disabled than one with a thoracic lesion; a patient with a thoracic lesion less disabled than one with a cervical lesion. The level of the lesion in the particular region is also significant.

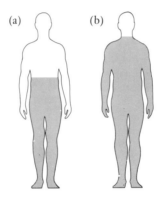

Fig. 5.1.   (a) Paraplegia; (b) Tetraplegia.

As each spinal nerve leaves the cord by two roots, one from the front and the other from the back of the spinal cord, it follows that some of the pathways from the anterior or posterior surface of the spinal cord may survive without interruption if the spinal cord is only partially transected. It is for this reason that some paraplegic patients may feel sensations in the skin and other tissues although their muscles are paralysed; the sensory pathways are intact but the motor pathways are interrupted.

Most paraplegic patients have paralysis of muscles and loss of sensation in skin, joints and bones below the level of transection of their spinal cord.

Usually there is also involvement of urinary bladder, bowel and rectum, genital organs and abdominal wall with the problems attendant upon paralysis of these structures.

Around the spinal cord there are nerve centres for the autonomic nervous system, both sympathetic and parasympathetic (Fig. 5.2). These are concerned with the visceral muscular control of the rectum and colon, the urinary bladder, the vasomotor system and the sexual organs. These parts are affected, resulting in loss of function, in some spinal lesions.

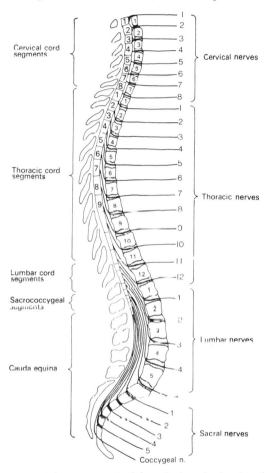

Fig. 5.2. The segmental arrangement of the spinal cord related to the spinal nerves.

THE CAUSES OF PARAPLEGIA

Traumatic

1 Road transport accidents. Today road transport accidents are responsible for the greatest percentage of paralysed patients.

2 Industrial accidents. To miners, dockers and building workers, either

by crushing injuries due to heavy weights falling on them, or by the worker falling from a height.

3 Sporting accidents such as a fall from a horse, or swimmers high diving into water too shallow to receive them.

4 Accidents in the home, such as falling down a flight of stairs.

Non-traumatic

Such cases are rare but may be classified as follows:

1 Congenital. Myelomeningocele and spina bifida. The infant is born with a defect both in the theca and the spinal cord (Fig. 5.3).

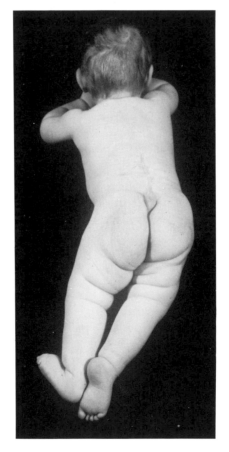

Fig. 5.3. Myelomeningocele and spina bifida. This infant was born with a defect in the theca and the spinal cord, but has had a corrective operation.

2 Deformities. Severe scoliosis and kyphosis (see Chapter 6), caused either by congenital or acquired lesions which may progress to paraplegic unless effectively treated (Fig. 5.4).

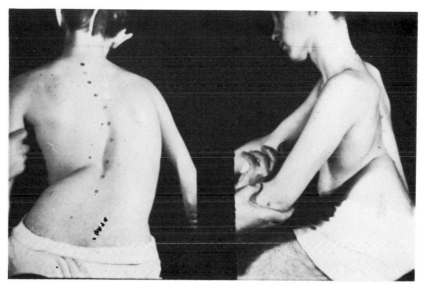

Fig. 5.4. Severe scoliotic and kyphotic deformities resulting in paraplegia.

3 Degenerative conditions; multiple sclerosis; scarring and fibrosis of various areas in the central nervous system.

4 Transverse myelitis; a section of the cord is destroyed and replaced by scar tissue probably because of a virus infection (Fig. 5.5).

Infections

Tuberculosis can affect the central nervous system. It may take the form either of tuberculous meningitis (inflammation of the meninges) or Pott's paraplegia (pressure on the spinal cord due to the presence of the products of a tuberculous abscess). (Fig. 5.6a, b).

Vascular

Arteriosclerosis may affect the spinal cord; it takes the form of progressive ischaemia until the spinal cord dies and its nerve fibres are replaced by a special type of fibrous scar tissue called gliosis.

Bleeding into the substance of the cord may also occur; this may be caused by trauma of disease.

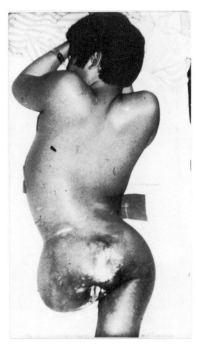

Fig. 5.5. Paraplegia due to transverse myelitis at level T_3-T_4 eleven years before this picture was taken. The patient is shown suffering from paralytic scoliosis.

Neoplasm

Primary tumours may occur either in the membranes or the bone surrounding the brain and spinal cord, resulting in compression and constriction of the cord.

Secondary tumours from carcinoma elsewhere in the body may arise in the vertebrae and in other tissues adjacent to the spinal cord (Fig. 5.7).

Relevant first aid in spinal injuries

The results of mismanagement of patients who sustain a fracture-dislocation of the spinal column can be awesome and irrevocable. Therefore as a first aid measure, it is wiser to treat every patient with the slightest suspicion of spinal injury as if he has a severe injury until proven otherwise by medical examination and radiography. Relatively slight injuries (whiplash injuries to the neck in a transport accident, for example) can cause permanent paralysis of the whole body without any sign of a wound or bruising. It is always best to assume that the neck or spine is fractured and dislocated when lifting and transporting these patients.

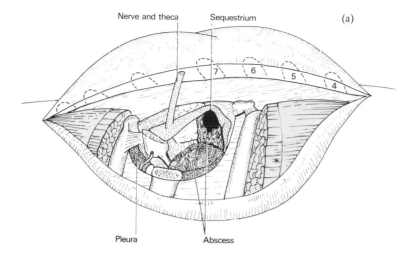

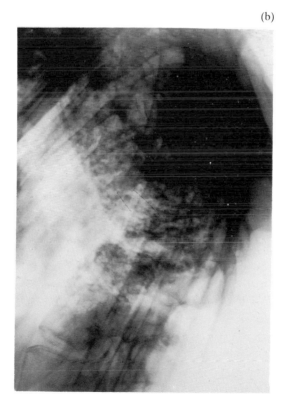

Fig. 5.6. (a) A tuberculous abscess compressing the spinal cord; (b) A radiograph of a tuberculous spine, with paraplegia.

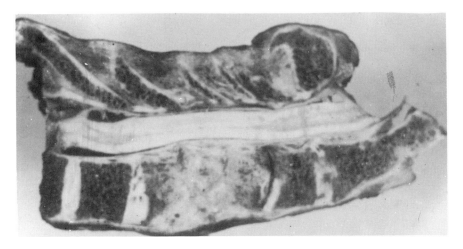

Fig. 5.7. A vertebral tumour compressing the spinal cord.

METHODS OF LIFTING

The patient can only be lifted by a number of people—four to six—working as a team. Rather than one or two persons attempting to raise the patient from the ground it is better to cover him until more help can be obtained. A strong blanket or sheet is used to lift the patient.

The patient must be carefully rolled, slowly and evenly, by the team with the head and neck carefully aligned to the rest of the body by one member of the team who concentrates on this sole function throughout the procedure. The helper at the head is opposed by a person at the feet who pulls the ankles and legs to help maintain the patient's body straight. The ankles and knees should be fastened together. (Fig. 5.8).

Before moving the patient a blanket is rolled lengthwise for two-thirds of its width. When the team have rolled the patient towards one side, the roll of the blanket is placed on the ground under him. The patient's body rolled back across the roll and over to the other side when the roll of blanket is then drawn through to the opposite side. The blanket is then used to lift the patient evenly from the ground while a board or stretcher is slipped under the blanket and the patient; at least three people to each side are necessary for this procedure. (Fig. 5.9).

Supports to the head in the form of a sandbag or small pillow at either side, and soft rolls of padding in the hollows behind the neck and lumbar spine are helpful in restricting movement of the patient's spine (Fig. 5.10).

The patient should be moved to hospital with care to avoid severe

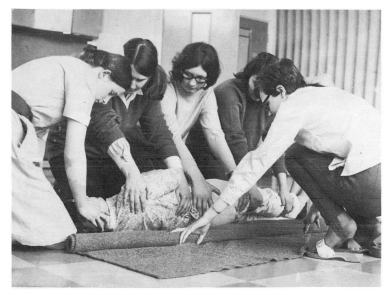

Fig. 5.8. Rolling a patient with a suspected spinal injury. The rolled blanket is placed under the patient and he is lifted on to it

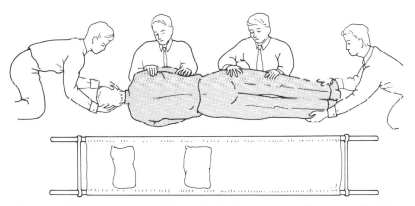

Fig. 5.9. The correct way to lift a spinal injuries patient. The patient is rolled onto a blanket or stretcher with longitudinal traction on head and legs.

jolting. The same careful, slow, but firm handling must, of course, be continued on arrival.

The pathology of acute lesions of the spinal cord

Damage to the spinal cord is usually, but not invariably, associated with damage to the spinal column. One must therefore consider both the

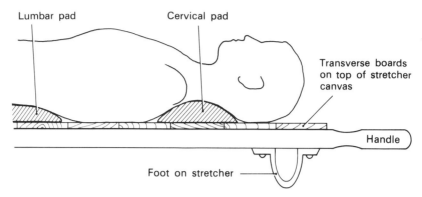

Fig. 5.10. Patient lying on a firm base with lumbar and cervical pillows. This is the correct method to support spinal injuries patients.

pathological changes due to injuries to the spinal column and the pathological changes in the spinal cord. It must of course, be recognized that in many instances, damage to the spinal cord occurs at the moment of injury and is often complete and irreversible; therefore, treatment of the spinal column itself, does not necessarily, indeed usually does not lead to any improvement in spinal cord function. On the other hand, if there has been minimal or no damage to the spinal cord and there is an unstable spinal fracture or dislocation, then failure to treat this may lead to subsequent irreversible damage to the partially damaged or undamaged spinal cord. In addition, in the rehabilitation of the patient, after a complete spinal transection the restoration of stability, integrity and strength to the spine is usually of considerable importance.

Injuries to the spinal column have been classified in a variety of ways. One mode of classification between stable and unstable conditions. Unfortunately, these terms are slightly ambiguous. In a strictly physical sense, any object is stable or is in equilibrium when the total sum of the forces, that is displacing and rotatory forces acting on it in all three dimensions, add up to zero, but of course, the normal spine moves. Therefore a spine can be perfectly normal and stable and yet the forces acting on a given vertebra may be causing it to move. At that moment, the spine is in the strict sense not in physical equilibrium and the sum of forces does not add up to zero. Accordingly one must modify, the strict physical definition of stability by defining stability as occurring when at the end of a physiological movement, the sum of forces acting on a segment of the spine returns to zero.

This definition is relevant because one might have sustained for instance, a minor crush fracture of the spine, which is usually regarded as being completely stable, and yet if the same patient were to sustain a further major fall, this might render the spine unstable and cause further damage, i.e. unphysiological forces have made it unstable. Nevertheless, for practical purposes, one can distinguish between those lesions of the spinal column in which there is a considerable risk of further displacement, and those in which there is a minimal risk. Equally, experience teaches us that certain types of lesions of the spinal column are usually associated with complete and irreversible damage to the spinal cord while other types of lesion are associated with either no damage or with partial or transient damage. The classical example of the latter category is of course, a simple compression fracture usually whether this is in the cervical, thoracic or lumbar region, there is no, or only transient or partial damage to the spinal cord. Because there is no tearing of ligaments or dislocation of joints, the spine is perfectly stable and minimal orthopaedic treatment is required. But there are severe compression fractures, the worst of which are often termed bursting fractures. In these the force applied to the spine is very much greater, the vertebral body is completely disintegrated. These fractures are usually associated with severe damage to the spinal cord and with considerable instability. Unless steps are taken to restore stability there will be progressive kyphosis and perhaps later, subluxation of the posterior articulations.

Other types of injury of the spine which are often combined are rotatory and lateral flexion injuries (Fig. 5.11). These are associated with dislocation of one posterior spinal articulation or alternatively, fracture of an articular process. These commonly occur both in the cervical and in the thoraco-lumbar regions; in the cervical region, they are usually accompanied by only partial damage to the spinal cord or perhaps damage to a nerve root. In the thoraco-lumbar region they are often accompanied by severe damage

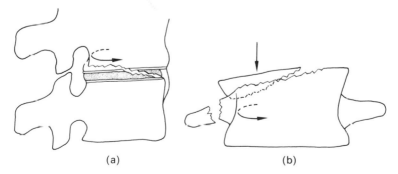

(a)   (b)

Fig. 5.11.   A lateral rotatory and flexion injury of the vertebral column.

to the lower part of the spinal cord and often complete and irreversible paraplegia. Complete dislocations of both posterior articulations are usually due to a horizontally displacing force and are nearly always accompanied by severe and often complete disruption of the spinal cord, but on occasions, such injuries are seen without major neurological damage. In these circumstances, it is extremely important to prevent further displacement and further damage occurring to the spinal cord.

Finally, one may have lesions of the spinal column due to a hyper-extension or what is sometimes called, a deflexion force, that is, excessive bending back of the spinal column with rupture of the anterior longitudinal ligament and often partial damage to the spinal cord.

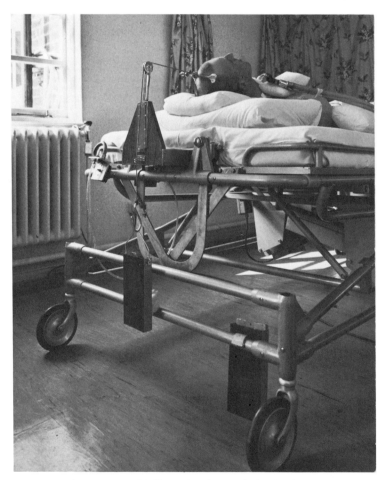

Fig. 5.12(a). Skull traction for cervical spine injury.

It is not within the scope of this book to discuss all possible types of injury of the spinal column, and all possible treatments; but one might summarize by saying that unstable fractures, or fracture dislocations of the cervical spine are usually best treated by a period of skeletal traction in recumbency (Fig. 5.12a and b). If there has been dislocation of posterior articulations it is usually advisable to try to reduce these if the patient is seen within 48 hours of his injury. In a case of injuries to the spine at a lower level, the best treatment is usually simple posturing in recumbency by means of properly arranged pillows, the patient being nursed in a turning bed if he has loss of sensation.

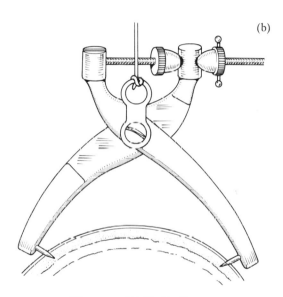

(b)

Fig. 5.12. (b) Skull calipers.

Pathological changes in the spinal cord

For obvious reasons we know little of the pathology of transient or incomplete lesions of the spinal cord. Post-mortem examination of irrecoverable lesions, shortly after injury, usually shows multiple scattered areas of haemorrhage and extensive tearing of cord substance. At a later date there will be atrophy and gliosis and possibly also cyst formation.

The role of such concepts as oedema and temporary ischaemia in transient paralysis is purely speculative.

In the case of hyperextension injuries with rupture of the anterior longitudinal ligament the patient merely needs nursing with the affected part of the spine held in slight flexion by some simple means such as a sorbo rubber collar (Fig. 5.13) or proper arrangement of pillows. In general,

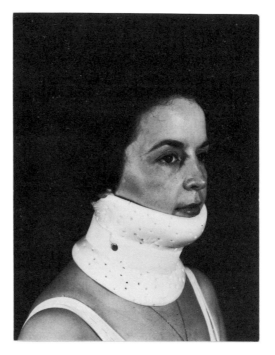

Fig. 5.13. A collar used in the management of hyperextension injuries in the cervical area.

it can be said that there is little, if any, role for laminectomy in the treatment of spinal column injuries associated with damage to the spinal cord, for the simple reason that the operative intervention will usually still further impair the stability of the spine. Also, in a badly shocked, injured patient, often with respiratory difficulty, it is inadvisable to subject them to operation unless it is clear that the operation is life-saving and will do the patient a considerable amount of good. For instance, if there is an associated rupture of a major viscous or associated severe injuries to the chest wall or diaphragm, these may require operative intervention to save the patient's life.

On the vexed question of the role of operative fixation of the spine, either with plates, wires or bone grafts, it can be said that the overwhelming majority of spinal injuries, that is, injuries to the spinal column, ultimately become perfectly stable by purely conservative treatment and the indications for intervention are relatively rare. As already indicated, in the overwhelming majority of cases, paralysis associated with injury to the spinal column is due either to complete rupture and tearing of the long tracts of the spinal cord, to a haematoma and scattered haemorrhages throughout the spine or to damage to blood vessels causing thrombosis and ischaemia of a part of the spine. In all these instances, it is very unlikely that any operative intervention will restore function to the damaged spine. Even when the spinal cord damage is partial but in the next day or two becomes worse, (often due to a transient ischaemia) there is no evidence that operative intervention with improve the prognosis. In complete paraplegia associated with injury to the spinal column, there is very little place for laminectomy or for immediate operative fixation of the spine. There may, however, be varying instances where the spine remains unstable and at a later date operative stabilization by some procedure such as bone grafting may be desirable. Perhaps one exception to this is where there is an injury to the lower part of the lumbar spine with a complete cauda equina lesion. In such circumstances there may be a role for laminectomy if the cauda equina nerves have not been disrupted but have merely been pressed upon by a displaced fragment of bone or a portion of disc material. Therefore, if the injury is in the lumbar spine and affecting the cauda equina only, it will be reasonable to perform an immediate myelogram. If there is evidence of a complete block, an operation should be performed to relieve this. Similarly, in very rare instances, where a portion of lamina has been driven inwards and is pressing on the spinal cord and this can be clearly demonstrated for example, by myelography, or tomograms, then there may be a place for operative removal. It must be stressed, however, that both of these are rather rare circumstances. The picture of paraplegia associated with spinal column injury may, of course, be complicated. Preceding disease of the spinal column, for example, a tumour or osteoporosis, or infection can precipitate a state of affairs which probably would have occured, anyway, but not as soon as with the trauma. Similarly, there may be a pre-existing disorder of the spinal cord for example, a tumour (especially a vascular tumour such as haemangioma) and a minor injury may precipitate a haemorrhage into such a tumour and cause paraplegia.

One must refer to the fact that in children it is possible to have a paraplegia secondary to an injury without there being any radiological evidence of major damage to the spinal column or myelographic evidence of a space-

occupying lesion. While the exact cause of such injuries is obscure, it
appears that they may be due to damage to the blood supply.

Lastly, under this heading, one must refer to instances where perhaps
two or three days after an operation such as a laminectomy or spinal fusion
the patient gradually loses spinal cord function and may become completely paraplegic. It appears that in the majority of instances there has
been a slow progressive thrombosis of one of the important arteries such as
the artery of Adamkiewicz which supplies the spinal cord. This, of course,
is one of the hazards of any operation of the thoracic or thoraco-lumbar
spine, however skilfully done. The surgeon may damage an important blood
vessel which may lead to subsequent loss of cord function. Many surgeons
advocate almost as a routine operation as plating, wiring or bone grafting
of the spine for a wide variety of injuries on the grounds that this obviates
the risk of later deformity and the development of neurological signs at a
later date. It is true that occasionally, many years after an injury, there may
be some signs of neurological deterioration. This is particularly true after
injuries in the upper cervical region, for instance, a fracture of the odontoid
process or an atlanto-axial dislocation. If such injuries fail to become stable
with conservative means, there certainly is a place for operative stabilization.
But at either level in the spine, such late deterioration is extremely rare
indeed so rare that it hardly justifies the risks and unpleasantnesses of what,
in 99 out of 100, is a quite unnecessary major operation. The late deterioration due to progressive instability of the spinal column must of course, be
distinguished from another type of late deterioration which occurs following
spinal injuries due to progressive syringomyelia usually associated with
ischaemia of the spinal cord. In this case the cause of the deterioration is
almost certainly vascular insufficiency and is not a direct mechanical con-
sequence of any real or fancied instability of the spine. This does not imply
that the stability of the spinal column is unimportant. Indeed, in the rehabilitation of a patient with complete paraplegia, spinal stability and good
control by muscle development is of the greatest possible importance. Severe
deformity is a great disadvantage to the patient and may lead to difficulty
in his rehabilitation, ability to sit, manoeuvre his wheelchair, etc. On the
other hand, fixation of a long segment of the spine as is necessary if the
spine is stabilized by a plate, may be still more deleterious to his rehabilitation. Such operations have a fairly high complication rate because plates
break, screws cut out or become loose, spinal processes break or infection
occurs in any considerable series. It has frequently been found necessary
to remove a plate which has been used for fixation and found to be relatively
ineffective or, alternatively, too effective, i.e. too long a segment is made

rigid. The idea that plating of the spine would make early rehabilitation easier has not in general been supported by the hard facts of clinical experience.

Examination of a spinal injury

The examination of a patient immediately after spinal injury is of course, of paramount importance. Spinal injuries may be associated with damage to the head, the cranial nerves, the thorax, the abdomen or the limbs. General examination will include the above with special emphasis on the patient's level of consciousness, blood pressure, pulse rate, respiratory rate and colour.

Clinical examination of the spine includes inspection for deformity, cuts, abrasions and bruises and palpation for any possible malalignment or separation of spinous processes. Examination of the limbs for voluntary power and sensibility must include marking the level below which these functions are lost. Examination of reflex function is of less assistance at this stage.

Results of damage

EARLY

Spinal shock may be the immediate result of damage to the spinal cord. All the segments of the cord below the point of injury cease to function. The urinary bladder loses its power to contract and skin sensations cannot be felt. The muscles receiving a nerve supply from that segment cannot be moved and are flaccid and flabby without muscle tone. The rectum and sexual organs are also similarly affected.

Spinal chock is often transient and a degree of recovery or sometimes even complete recovery may occur if there has not been significant permanent damage to nerve cells.

LATER

After recovery from spinal shock, any paralysis remaining is permanent and residual. Although optimism is the keynote of paraplegic management, the attitudes of the patient and his relatives must be directed towards acceptance of the existing paralysis of the patient, and modification of his way of life to meet the new situation. Some recovery does occur much later in a few patients, but this is not a common occurence.

Problems of paraplegia and tetraplegia

Classification

Pain
Spasm
Respiratory failure, acute or chronic
Loss of urinary control
Urinary infection
Loss of bowel control
Constipation
Loss of sexual function
Loss of sensation
Vulnerability to burns and other injuries
Decubitus ulcers
Loss of movement in limbs
Psychological distress
Loss of occupation and earnings

PAIN

Pain will usually be the result of the initial injury. A later serious problem however, is 'root pain' which is due to irritation of the affected nerve roots. This does not affect all patients but is a great trial to those it does affect. It presents serious problems for the doctor responsible for the patient, as the drugs provided must be carefully chosen in the light of the other problems of paraplegia.

SPASM

Once the segment of the cord below the point of transection has recovered from spinal shock, it functions in a normal way but, being detached from the brain it can receive no instructions by the normal pathways and works independently. One pathway which is broken normally inhibits the reflex arc. This is a local phenomenon of muscle contraction dependent on a segment of the cord and a set of muscles. It uses the spinal nerve as a connecting link. The absence of inhibition from the brain means that the reflex arc acts independently, erratically and with minimal stimulation. Thus, irritation of the skin or a full bladder, constipation or emotion can cause the paralysed limbs of the patient to contract forcefully. The contractions are usually accompanied by rhythmical shaking of the affected limbs.

Apart from the inconvenience for the patient and his attendants, such spasms may result in sores as the skin of the limbs is rubbed against the opposite limb and on other surfaces.

Because the reflex arc is intact the muscles of the limbs do not waste so much as in paralysis due to peripheral nerve lesions; muscle tone is present and is usually excessive. Treatment of this problem may take the following forms:

1 Relieving the cause of the spasm if it can be found. Distension of bowel or bladder are obvious examples.

2 Nursing measures to hold the affected limbs and prevent them from going into spasm.

3 Physiotherapy: application of heat and massage to the affected muscles; passive movements to prevent contractures of joint capsules and muscles.

4 Surgical means such as tenotomy, neurectomy or interruption of the reflex arc.

RESPIRATORY FAILURE

Acute. Soon after the injury, the patient may have difficulty in breathing if the level of his lesion is high enough up the spinal cord to involve the thorax. Later, an ascending paralysis may increasingly affect the chest and even the diaphragm. Regurgitation of stomach contents may also occur as part of the initial injury with inhalation of the vomit from the mouth.

Chronic. Efficient coughing requires the full use of the abdominal and thoracic muscles. If the abdominal walls are paralysed it is difficult for the patient to expel air from the thorax and secretions from the trachea and bronchi.

In patients with any paralysis of the abdomen, diaphragm or thorax, breathing is inefficient and mucous secretions gather in the bronchioles and obstruct repiratory efforts still further. Such patients are liable to chest infections.

Help may take the following forms:

1 Careful observation of patients with cervical lesions. They must not be left unattended, particularly during the acute stages.

2 The use of mechanical ventilators for patients with a cervical lesion.

3 Tracheostomy to assist the intermittent positive pressure ventilation provided by a mechanical ventilator, and to help evacuation of the respiratory passages by suction.

4 Assisted coughing; the nursing or physiotherapy staff apply pressure to the thorax and abdomen of the patient to help. Later, if possible, the patient compresses his own abdomen during coughing.

URINARY PROBLEMS

During the phase of spinal shock, urine is at first retained in the urinary bladder which distends. When the limit of distension has been reached, the urine overflows, resulting in passive incontinence. This may last for a few hours or some days.

When the detached segment of the spinal cord recovers and is able to resume its activity, the bladder may return to the primitive ('reflex') function present in the young infant; in this state it contracts and empties as its walls are stretched. This creates an intermittent complete evacuation of urine. The management of the patient's condition may include training the patient to estimate the intervals between emptying so that he may arrange a toilet programme. Many patients learn to evacuate the bladder when they desire to do so by compressing the pubic area of the abdomen with the hand.

A major problem for every paraplegic or tetraplegic patient is the possibility of infection of the urinary tract with resultant serious illness. Until recently urinary infections and resulting renal failure was the most common cause of death in paraplegics. Management of these urinary problems are discussed more fully later in this chapter (page 139).

BOWEL PROBLEMS

As a result of division of sensory tracts the patient is unaware of the contents of his rectum. Additionally, the absence of muscle tone in the bowel and rectum retards normal colonic actions and slows the normal forward movement of faeces and flatus.

Distension of the abdomen, digestive distress and constipation are paraplegic problems. These are discussed fully later in this chapter.

LOSS OF SEXUAL FUNCTION

Paralysis of the genital organs means that normal sexual function is not possible. The female paraplegic patient may become pregnant, however. This inability to reproduce and probably to remain unmarried is a cause of major psychological distress in many younger male paraplegic patients.

LOSS OF SENSATION OF SKIN FUNCTION

The paralysed patient with damage to the sensory nerves or tracts will have no sensation in the skin of the affected parts. This creates problems of temperature regulation for the patient as well as making him unaware of danger from burning or other hazards to his person. Such hazards as fires, radiators or exposure to severe cold with frostbite are to be avoided.

Related to this is the problem of poor muscle and skin tone. Prolonged unrelieved pressure on the tissues may not be felt and will result in the breakdown of the skin with necrotic ulceration, ultimately progressing to deep craters if untreated. Infection and anaemia may increase the problem.

The patient must be on his guard to prevent decubitus ulcers for the rest of his life.

LOSS OF NORMAL MOBILITY

This problem creates severe frustration for the patient who cannot now do the things he could before his accident. This is most serious in a person who was used to leading an active life in sports and other activities; it calls for major mental and physical readjustment in all patients. In addition, the loss of mobility causes osteoporosis and a high renal excretion of calcium with a tendency to form urinary stones.

PSYCHOLOGICAL DISTRESS

In the initial phase of paralysis the patient will not accept that he will never walk normally again; When he sees others who are paralysed he thinks, 'I am different—it could not happen to me, I am going to recover.' Later, when his position becomes more obvious, he develops a severe mental depression. On recovery he may accept his lot and adapt to his new way of life.

The medical, nursing and physiotherapy staff must help him through the various stages of progression and create the optimism he requires for his rehabilitation. It is better if he is gently introduced to the inevitability of his state by graduated stages—a little information at a time.

LOSS OF OCCUPATION AND EARNINGS

A problem for any person who can no longer perform the work he has been trained to do is loss of earnings and thus dependence on welfare funds, compensation or charity.

A vigorous retraining and re-employment regime is undertaken for the paralysed person and many return to earning their living and paying income tax; but many do not.

The desire to earn and continue to support his family may provide the motivation to work for early rehabilitation.

Hospital management

The survival and rehabilitation of the paraplegic patient is more likely to occur in Spinal Injuries Units with teams of experienced specialist

workers to care for him. The fastest possible means should be used to transfer the patient; the ideal is by helicopter or ambulance collection from the
scene of the accident and direct admission to the spinal injuries centre.

In the Spinal Injuries Unit the special equipment and accommodation
required for spinal injuries patients is centralized.

The patients within the unit may be classified as follows:

1   Acute, new lesions, with the patients under intensive care. Those with
high lesions in the cervical area, will come into this group.

2   New lesions not under intensive care within 12 weeks of the initial
injury. There may be additional injuries to the spinal lesion.

3   Patients from category 1 or 2 who have progressed to a level of independence and are nearing discharge after rehabilitation.

4   Old lesions; patients re-admitted with problems such as decubitus
ulcers or for re-assessment and further rehabilitation.

Aims of management

The principal aim is to rehabilitate the patient in order that he may live in
normal home surroundings and to take up an occupation with minimal
dependence on others. These aims are ideals; many patients achieve them
but others do not. There are many complications to be avoided. The end
results of treatment depend upon the intelligence and motivation of the
patient. To assist him in his rehabilitation the consistent efforts of skilled
and conscientious members of the Spinal Injuries Unit are required.

The stages of management are:

1   resuscitation
2   reduction of the spinal lesion
3   prevention of complications
4   return to home and employment with independence

Immediate treatment

In the period immediately following admission to the unit the patient
will be ill—not only with his spinal injury but often with additional trauma
to other parts of his body. Severe limb, abdominal, thoracic or cranial
injuries may be present; there may be severe loss of blood; most certainly
the patient will be shocked and bewildered. The injuries, other than the
spinal injury, must be treated concurrently. The morale of the patient must
be maintained and the attitude of his nursing team is related. There must
be no disgust, revulsion or useless pity; the patient must be treated as a
person—as should any patient. High standards of personal hygiene and

grooming are important and must not be allowed to lapse, otherwise the patient will become dejected or ashamed. His mode of address by his proper name, Mr ——, is also essential.

The patient's bed

A conventional hospital bed is used with additional pillows or sorbo rubber pads (Fig. 5.14). These pillows are used, (a) to roll the patient in turning; (b) to prevent pressure on bony prominences and (c) to adjust the patient in the desired position.

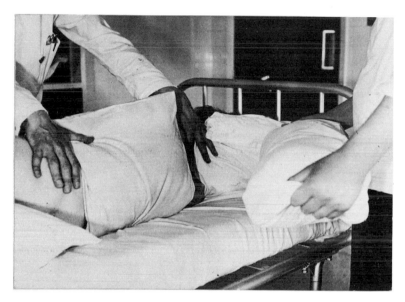

Fig. 5.14. Spinal support pillow on the bed of a spinal injuries patient.

A bed cradle, a bracket to support the urine receiving bag and a firm supporting pad for his feet which will maintain his ankles at a right angle are extra requirements. Electrically operated turning beds are also available (Fig. 5.15). A Stryker bed is sometimes used.

The clothing

In the early management of the patient he is nursed without clothing. This is the most convenient way during the period of intensive care as otherwise bladder, bowel and thoracic management would require constant undressing and re-dressing of the patient.

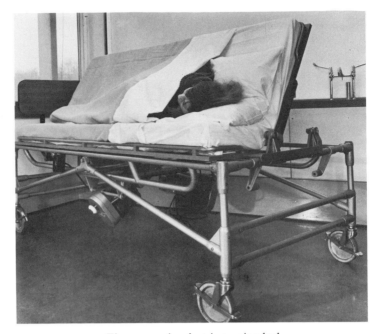

Fig. 5.15.   An electric turning bed.

THE POSITION OF THE PATIENT

The patient's position is altered by a steady relentless routine of two-hourly turning. Each turn is charted and is carried out at exactly the time stated both night and day. A nursing team of sufficient numbers must be provided to maintain this routine in every spinal injuries unit. Once the turning routine is established the patient will wake automatically and, if he has the use of his arms, will eventually be able to turn himself as rehabilitation progresses.

THE TURNING ROUTINE

When there is a shortage of nursing staff for turning the patient, devices such as electric turning beds have their place. When sufficient nurses can be assembled to turn the patient, however, the conventional bed with extra pillows is preferable.

Before turning, bedcovers, pillows and other accessories are removed to leave a clear field. The most experienced nurse stays at the head of the bed to control the head turning and any traction weights, cords and pulleys. She has a second function in giving clear and concise instructions to the other team members so that actions are in unisen. The turning routine is as follows:

(a) FROM SUPINE TO LATERAL

1   The leg away from the side to which the patient will turn is carried across the near leg.

2   The arms are arranged; they are best carried on the chest. If the patient can cooperate, he may fold his arms to control them.

3   The patient's body is carried over towards the side of the bed away from that which he will face on completion of the turn. A thin lumbar pillow which is in position in the hollow of the back is used to lift the trunk by two nurses, one on either side of the bed, who use the pillow as a sling to carry the patient. Another pair of nurses lift the legs and carry them over in line with the trunk. Care is taken to clear the buttocks of the patient from the undersheet so that the skin is not 'scuffed' as the patient is moved. During this move the nurse at the head carefully aligns the head and neck with trunk.

4   The patient is now rolled slowly and evenly in to the lateral position using the lumbar pillow as a device for rotating him.

5   The legs of the patient are now used to fix him in a stable position. The upper leg is placed straight down the bed on pillows with the ankle at a right angle. The lower leg is flexed at the hip, knee and ankle and adjusted so that the hip is flexed but neither abducted nor adducted.

6   The arms are placed comfortably so that they are not under the body. A pillow may be required to support the upper arm.

7   A bed cradle is placed over the patient's legs and the bed remade.

(b) FROM LATERAL TO SUPINE

1   At the start of the procedure the patient is rolled still further towards the prone position so that the undersheet and lumbar pillow may be checked and smoothed, or else replaced.

2   The patient is first rolled on to his back with the lumbar pillow held firmly against his spine; after this his body is lifted to the centre of the bed.

3   The legs are arranged with both hips partially flexed and abducted, both knees slightly flexed and both ankles at a right angle.

POSITIONING THE UPPER LIMBS

The turning routines described above are applied to all spinal injury patients even on head traction. A similar procedure is used for patients who are paraplegic or tetraplegic. In caring for any of these patients, a set routine of movement from right lateral to supine, and from supine to left lateral, at two-hourly intervals must be maintained during the whole twenty-four hours of the day. A chart of these turnings must be kept and entered by the staff who carry out each turn.

In the interim period whilst awaiting transfer to a spinal injuries unit from the initial hospital, probably the greatest contribution the nursing staff can make is to commence and establish a turning routine for the patient. If turning is not carried out, or even if missed for one routine, pressure sores will occur.

The positions used are standard and are considered the least likely to result in fixed deformity or pressure sores. The positions also contribute to the reduction of muscle spasm.

When the patient has paralysis of the upper limbs also special care is needed. Flexion contractures of the elbows and wrists should be avoided by placing them in extension. To avoid adduction contractures of the shoulders they should be arranged in abduction. The hands should be arranged around a roll or in special hand splints to avoid deformity of the fingers. The web between index finger and thumb should be at 'full-stretch'.

Prevention of decubitus ulcers

A catastrophe for any paralysed patient, whether new and acute, or old and chronic, is a decubitus ulcer. Such an ulcer can be deep, infected and sloughing. It can be complicated by involvement of a joint, bone or other important structure other than skin. Most of them take a considerable length of time to resolve and heal and all will retard the progression of the patient to rehabilitation and independence.

The problem of liability to ulcers usually exists because the patient feels no sensation in the areas which are vulnerable. He is unaware that a lesion exists until it is in an advanced stage. Another contributory factor is that the normal resistance to pressure, which exists in the unparalysed person is absent because of the vasomotor paralysis; there is no bone in the tissue.

Some patients may also have other contributory problems such as anaemia, emaciation or obesity. Spasticity in limbs is another factor in the creation of continued, unrelieved pressure on the tissues which ends in the breakdown and rupture of the superficial coverings of the body.

SITES OF DECUBITUS ULCERS

These will occur on any bony prominence when the bone presses hard against the mattress or other surface and deprives the skin, which is trapped in the pressure, of its blood supply. Thus all the spinous processes, the sacrum, the iliac crests, the iliac spines, the great trochanters of the femurs, the epicondyles of femurs, the condyles of tibiae, the malleoli, heels and feet are all vulnerable.

The patient who is seated in a wheelchair is liable to severe ulcers on the ischial tuberosities and the sacro-coccygeal area and must establish a 'press-up' reflex as soon as he transfers from bed to chair (Fig. 5.16).

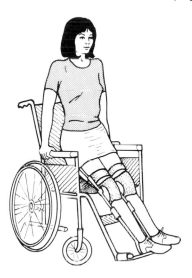

Fig. 5.16. A spinal injuries patient doing press-ups to avoid decubitus ulcers.

EDUCATION OF THE PATIENT

As soon as the patient is orientated to the fact that he is paralysed, and will probably always be, he must be made 'pressure-conscious'. This means that he must be made aware of what decubitus ulcers are (perhaps show him photographs) and how disastrously they can affect his independence and the means he can take to prevent them. These measures are:

1 Avoiding consistent relentless pressure on any part of his paralysed anatomy. This involves:

(a) whilst in bed the patient's position is changed to a timed routine (see page 128). At first this is done for him by attendants who conform to a pattern which is maintained during the whole twenty-four hours of the day. As he recovers and achieves some measure of independence he may learn to turn himself in his bed and imbues in himself a waking/turning reflex which does not require watches or clocks.

(b) whilst in a wheelchair he develops a reflex 'press-ups' routine so that, even without applying thought to his actions, he uses his upper limbs, (if he has the use of them) to elevate his buttocks and thighs from the base of the chair every ten minutes (Fig. 5.16).

2 Regular daily self-inspection of all likely areas for the formation of decubitus ulcers by the use of a reflecting mirror. If this is not feasible he must arrange to be inspected by an attendant. Reporting to his medical or nursing advisor the presence of any red area which does not clear, bruises, blisters, skin breaks, or swelling, as soon as possible after discovery.

3 Avoiding periods of irresponsibility resulting from intoxication.

4 Avoiding the danger of burns and scalds.

5 Maintaining his general health at its optimum level.

The nursing staff responsible for the patient confined to bed avoid turning the patient on to the surface which appears to be undergoing change towards ulceration. Thus if the great trochanter on one side is affected that side will not be involved in the turning routine.

The management of decubitus ulcers

As already stated (on page 130) decubitus ulcers are an avoidable catastrophe. The patient who is well trained in avoiding the causative pressure by carrying out 'press-ups' and otherwise varying position at frequent intervals, and is intelligent and physically fit enough to practice what has been taught will not acquire them. They *do* occur, however, and they then require the patient's re-admission to the spinal unit, return to bed and loss of acquired independence, and the probability of seriously reducing the level of physical fitness. The management of the patient, on return to the spinal unit is as follows:

1 Pressure is taken off the sore entirely by positioning the patient in the prone position (if there is a sacro-coccygeal sore, for example) and maintaining a turning routine which does not include the supine position.

2 Arranging a full clinical examination of the patient to exclude pathological conditions which may have caused the decubitus ulcer. A full blood chemistry and urinalysis is performed to exclude such diseases as diabetes mellitus, any of the anaemic or ischaemic conditions which might affect the equality of the tissues. Another factor to exclude is infection although it is a good principle to regard a decubitus ulcer as already infected.

3 Improving the physical state of the patient with intravenous, diet and pharmacological therapy. This means blood transfusion if needed, a therapeutic diet with a high content of protein, minerals and vitamins, and the administration of appropriate antibiotics, mineral elements and vitamins during the medication round.

4   Good general management of the patient by the spinal unit team to ensure that the patient does not deteriorate whilst bedfast.

5   A positive approach to the ulcer which includes:

(a)   Surgical toilet to remove ischaemic and necrotic material.

(b)   The use of desloughing agents such as Aserbine.

(c)   Frequent surgical dressings using bland detergent and solvent lotions. Packs may be necessary but these must be loosely arranged within the wound. The dressings are firmly positioned.

(d)   Skin grafting may be needed if healing by granulation does not include a good cover to the ulcer site.

(e)   Careful return to mobilization for the patient as soon as this is feasible.

Prevention of contractures

Joints in normal and healthy people have a full range of movements optimum to the function of the limb and the needs of the body. When some of the range of movement has gone because of tethering by soft tissue this is known as a 'contracture' (Fig. 5.17). A contracture may be caused by

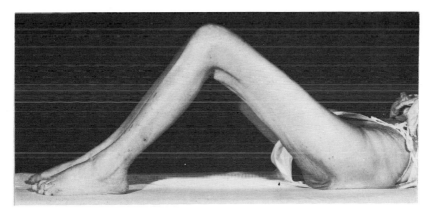

Fig. 5.17.   Flexion contractures in the limbs of a paralysed patient.

shortening, spasticity, loss of elasticity, or imbalance, of muscles and at-tached tendons or by changes in the structure of the joint capsule caused by disuse of the joint. They are most likely to occur in patients with neuro-logical disorders particularly when the muscle is served by a segment of spinal cord which is isolated from the main part of the central nervous system below a transection lesion. Contractures increase the problems of any paralysed patient. The presence of such contractures mean that the patient is unable to lie down or sit comfortably. The severe pressure of the skin and prominences of one limb against the other results in damage to skin and decubitus ulcer formation. A severely bent, contracted limb may also tremble when the patient is emotional or has a full bladder or bowel or has some other cause of distress.

It is not possible to prevent spasticity in limbs by nursing measures only. Pharmacological or surgical intervention is often necessary. Certain nursing measures can be applied to avoid contractures causing a permanent fixed deformity:

1　Efficient practical placing of the patients limbs related to the position of the body when supine, prone, left lateral or right lateral (page 129).

2　Regular systematic changing of the position of the patient and complete re-arrangement of the joint at each turn.

3　Tethering a contracted limb in an extended position by holding it in the fold of a sheet arranged around it and tucked firmly in below the mattress of the bed.

4　Using pillows arranged between the knees when a patient has an adduction spasm problem.

5　Vigorous physiotherapy to the affected joints.

6　Hydrotherapy in a heated pool.

7　Attempting to seek, find and treat the cause of any contracture.

Toilet routine

As already stated, the morale of the patient will be improved by the maintenance of a high level of personal hygiene. He will perspire heavily; be either incontinent of urine and faeces or require help to micturate and defaecate. A daily blanket bath is necessary and the genital and anal area must be kept clean by frequent washing. Shaving, hair washing and combing, oral hygiene and manicure for fingers and toes are all good points of patient care.

The skin of the paralysed legs and feet will require special attention. As the skin is not in normal use it becomes dry, hard and scaly.

Hard layers of dead epithelium which collects on the feet should be removed and the skin washed clean and a skin lotion with a lanolin content used to soften the underlying skin.

Diet. In the early stages a light nutritious diet is probably all that can be achieved. The most important diet content is that of fluid. Copious intake of all forms of fluids is a necessary part of the maintenance of kidney function and the prevention of renal failure. The vitamin and mineral content must be adequate.

As the patient progresses the diet content must be increased to about 2,000 calories per day. If the patient has any pressure sores and is losing serum and protein, the intake of protein must be increased accordingly.

As soon as possible the patient with full use of the upper limbs must be encouraged to feed himself; this may be difficult whilst lying supine but it is a skill which must be acquired.

The tetraplegic patient must be fed. To ensure an adequate intake frequent small nutritious meals are more suitable than large quantities at longer intervals. The person feeding the patient must sit down and give an unhurried impression; he need not be a nurse—visitors, relatives, voluntary helpers and non-nursing staff can all help, particularly in a unit where there are several patients who are totally paralysed.

An important content of the patient's diet is roughage. The approach to establishing a pattern of regular defaecation with minimal assistance will require an adequate amount of cellulose and cereal in the diet.

Extra protein in the diet may be provided as meat or cheese, or other dairy produce, but powdered protein may be required for some patients to ensure a large enough intake.

When some paralysis of the upper limbs exists there will be difficulty in lifting food from the plate and transferring it to the mouth. The occupational therapist will contribute by providing devices such as those shown in (Fig. 5.18) and training the patient in their method of use.

MANAGEMENT OF DEFAECATION

Because the patient is unaware of the contents of his colon he cannot know when defaecation is required. The abdominal muscles and colon walls contribute to the act of defaecation and as these are completely paralysed, they do not contribute much to the act of expelling either faeces or flatus. Pressure and massage by the hands on the abdomen may be necessary.

The process of evacuation of the bowel depends upon a regularly timed routine each day.

In the early bed management of the patient this habit must be established and a bowel action is caused at the same time each day. Ideally, before progression to a sitting or standing position, the patient's bowel routine should have become fixed at a definite time of day.

This bowel action should ideally be a natural process which can be achieved if all the factors related are considered.

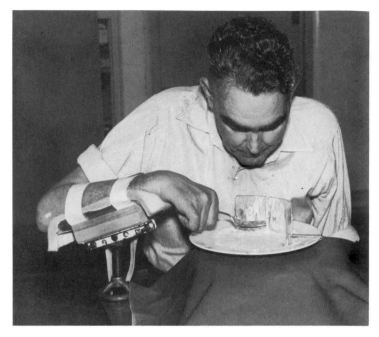

Fig. 5.18.   Devices used to assist the patient with upper-limb paralysis to feed himself.

1   *The diet content.* From the earliest days of management, roughage must be included in the food of the patient.

2   *The fluid intake.* This must be higher than was previously acceptable from both bowel and urinary consideration.

3   *Accurate timing.* A time schedule means that the patient will prepare for bowel evacuation even though the patient cannot feel the contents of his bowel.

4   *An awareness of distension.* Flatus in the bowel usually means that faeces are also present.

5   *The use of vegetable laxatives and faecal softeners.* Peristalsis is increased if a suitable laxative is provided. If the patient is having difficulties, laxatives are supplied in the evening in preparation for bowel evacuation the next day.

6   *Toilet training.* At first the patient will empty his bowel onto incontinence pads, but when he can be raised from his bed to a wheelchair he can use the ward lavatory—where an inflatable ring cushion to cover the seat must be available. A reflecting mirror on the wall at the back of the lavatory

above the level of the inflated ring seat is an asset. Lavatories with adequate door width and cubicle width to accommodate the wheelchair must be part of the unit; suitable devices for the patient to use to transfer himself independently onto the lavatory from his wheelchair are supplied; a supporting rail attached to the wall near the washdown closet is helpful. There must be no rush or hurry, although once the patient has established his own pattern he will require less time for the process.

7   *Suitable clothing*. Once the patient reaches independence when going on the lavatory, special clothing which can easily be removed is necessary. The aim is that the patient will pass a soft malleable bowel content with minimal difficulty at a set time each day.

8   Food taken before the bowel action is due will often stimulate colonic peristalsis.

9   Self-palpation of the abdomen may be helpful.

10 A full and deep inspiration may cause increased rectal pressure.

CONSTIPATION

Either constipation or diarrhoea are a problem for the patient. Constipation may be dealt with:

1   By the provision of a laxative.

2   By the use of a laxative suppository thirty minutes prior to the anticipated time of defaccation. In the early training the suppository must be used routinely.

3   Enemata. This is less desirable than the suppository because it may cause prolonged and repeated small bowel evacuation instead of a single movement. The small disposable enemata are preferable. When the faeces are hard and impacted 300 ml of warmed arachis or olive oil may be inserted thirty minutes prior to the purgative enema.

4   Manual interference. This is the least desirable method as it tends to dilate the anus and rectum so that any tonus in the muscle is lost. It must only be used as a last resort.

A lubricated rubbergloved finger is inserted into the bowel and any scybala are helped out with the crooked finger.

There is a danger, if constipation is not noted and reported and action is taken, that the patient may become obstructed, requiring advanced surgical assistance to overcome the problem.

Charting of bowel action time and amount is necessary for the bed patient.

Urinary bladder regime for paraplegic patients

INITIAL REGIME

(a)   *During the first twelve hours after the injury to the spine.*
    No attempt to catheterize or extract urine from the patient.

(b)   *After twelve hours when there are signs of bladder distension.*
    Catheterize the patient at eight-hourly intervals until some recovery from spinal shock when reflex emptying of the bladder can be achieved by the patient and less than 100 ml of urine remain.
    This latter fact is established by passing a catheter.

(c)   *When residual urine estimation shows a decrease.*
    Increase the interval between catheterization first to twelve hours and secondly every twenty-four hours and finally cease catheterization except for residual urine estimation on every third day.

(d)   *Other relevant nursing management.*
    During the early states after spinal injury there may be impaired urinary function. Oliguria is the major sign of this. During this phase the fluid intake may need to be reduced upon the instructions of the doctor in charge.

2   When this phase has passed the fluid intake of the patient must be increased to as large a quantity as possible, preferably when micturition will not disturb the sleep of the patient.

3   Careful recording of fluid intake and output and the daily balance must be maintained.

4   Pathological examination of the urine of the patient is necessary, frequently, and particularly if there are any signs of urinary infection.

LATER URINARY REGIME

    The functioning of the urinary bladder in the spinal lesion patient is related to the level of transection.

High level lesions

    In patients with a high level injury (cervical and upper thoracic) the cord below the level of the division is whole and intact and the nerves connecting the spinal cord to the bladder function as normally but without the controlling instructions from the brain. It is possible to establish the same reflex bladder activity which is present in an infant before toilet habits are instituted. When the bladder is filled, or partly filled, it is possible to cause an outflow of urine by stimulation of the musculature of the bladder wall so that it contracts and empties. Tapping the abdominal wall is an example of such a form of stimulation, but each patient will develop his or her own.

Lumbar and cauda equina lesions

In low spinal cord lesions there is an interference with the nerves communicating between the spinal cord and the urinary bladder and its sphincters and contraction muscles. This is in fact a form of peripheral nerve lesion with many of the effects referred to in Chapter 3. These include flaccidity and wasting of muscle tissue. In some of these patients it may be necessary for the urologist to intervene to assist the retention of urine within the bladder by altering the structure of the urethral sphincter. The bladder may be regarded as an inelastic bag which is emptied by being 'squashed' by firm abdominal pressure with the hands. At first this is done by attendants but eventually the patient must learn to do it himself. The interval between expulsion of urine is related to the volume of fluid drunk by the patient and the intelligent patient can regulate visits to the toilet by adjusting fluid intake to arrange two- or three-hourly intervals.

In either the high-level or low-level lesion patient surgical intervention by the urologist may be necessary or there may be no alternative but recourse to condom devices and drainage tubes and bags (Fig. 5.19) in the male patient or the making of an ileal bladder (see page 163) in the female patient. If either of these methods can be avoided by consistent competent training from the earliest post-trauma day possible the patient's enjoyment of a dry, confident, wheelchair existence is more assured.

URINARY INFECTION

The patient with a urinary infection can be very ill. Apart from the local signs of an infected bladder and urine, foul smelling, turbid, flocculent urine the patient will demonstrate all the signs of symptoms of any generalized infection: he feels unwell, loses his appetite, has nausea and may vomit, looks feverish and has a raised temperature, pulse and respiratory rate, and may be irritable and confused. Irrational atypical behaviour is often the first sign that something is wrong.

If the patient's urinary tract becomes infected his progress towards rehabilitation will be seriously retarded; reflex automatic bladder control may not be possible. However, good nursing techniques can prevent infection.

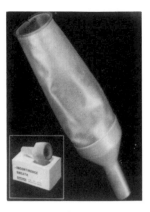

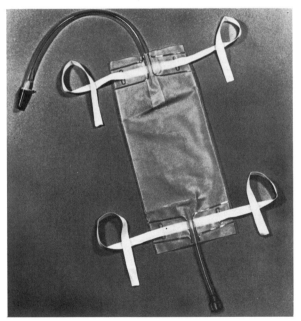

Fig. 5.19.   (a) Condom device for the incontinent male paraplegic. (b) Drainage tube and collecting bag for urine.

The complications of urinary infection

1   Pyelonephritis.
2   Urinary failure.
3   Inflammation of the ureters, urinary bladder and urethra with scar tissue formation and strictures.

4   Epididymo-orchitis occurs as the infection tracks along the vas deferens to the testicles of the male.

5   Generalized illness.

6   Secondary infection elsewhere in the body.

CATHETERS

(a)   *Red rubber catheters of the Jacques, Harris or Tiemann's type.* Such catheters are of value in intermittent catheterization—that is, the catheter is taken out of the urethra as soon as the procedure is completed. They are not suitable for fixing in the bladder as indwelling catheters, as they tend to irritate the lining of the urethra.

(b)   *Latex rubber catheters of the balloon type.* These catheters offer a wide lumen for drainage when large amounts of debris are present. The balloon is inflated within the bladder with 5 ml saline and this protuberance serves to hold the catheter inside the urethra. The latex rubber is less irritating than red rubber.

(c)   *Fine plastic catheters of the Gibbon type.* These are of much smaller external circumference than the lining of the urethra and are less likely to irritate to the medical side of the thigh of the female, using waterproof zinc oxide plaster. They are ideal provided the urine does not contain debris as they can easily become blocked.

(d)   *Silastic catheters.* This is an indwelling balloon catheter. It has the advantage of being non-irritant and may be left *in situ* for many weeks without changing. There is every reason to consider the silastic catheter as a useful addition to equipment needed in the management of the bladder of a paralysed patient.

HYGIENE OF THE PATIENT WITH AN INDWELLING CATHETER

The genitalia of either the male or female patient must be maintained scrupulously clean at all times. Thorough washing of the parts at least twice daily or when they become soiled is necessary. When an excessive amount of pubic hair is present this should be clipped.

Devices for collecting urine from the ambulant patient

There are several excellent devices for collection of urine into a portable receptacle available for the male patient (see Fig. 5.19b) but the female genital organs are not suitably shaped for the attachment of devices to facilitate urinary drainage. It may be necessary to help the incontinent female paraplegic patient by surgical means as described in the next paragraph, although some female patients manage with an indwelling catheter.

Ileal loop bladder for the female paraplegic patient

The female patient is provided by surgical means with an artificial bladder formed from a detached segment of the small intestine. The two ureters are detached from their lower insertion into the bladder and re-attached to the loop of intestine; this loop opens onto the anterior abdominal wall in a similar fashion to a colostomy or ileostomy opening. (Fig. 5.20). Thus the urinary bladder is by-passed and no urine passes through the urethra. A device can now be attached to the anterior abdominal wall to receive urine and keep the patient dry. This operation is specially useful if there is chronic incurable bladder infection.

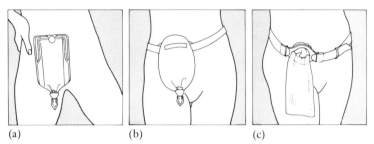

(a)   (b)   (c)

Fig. 5.20.   Three types of ileostomy bags on the anterior abdomen wall (see also Fig. 6.7).

Hygiene of the receptacles

As these receive urine they soon become fetid unless properly cleaned. The patient must have at least two and preferably three. The reserve urinal is cleaned carefully with detergent and antiseptic, dried, and hung up to allow air to reach the inside. Disposable equipment is preferable.

An essential factor for the self-esteem of the patient is the knowledge that the receptacle is reliable and will not let him down.

Management of condom devices

Disposable urinary incontinence devices are available. These consist of condoms, polythene tubing, connecting pieces, and polythene receptacle-bags (see Fig. 5.19) which are in use for a limited time and then discarded. They are obviously preferable to the non-disposable type which require much care and maintenance.

The condom

This is supplied by the manufacturers with a short length of latex tube attached to it. The condom device has the advantage, for the male patient, that it is less necessary to insert a catheter up the urethra and into the bladder with the possible hazard of introducing urinary infection.

Method of application

The penis of the patient must be clean and dry before the application of the condom and is washed and dried when the device is changed. A small amount of skin-adhesive is applied in a ring around the base of the penis and the condom is rolled on to above the level of the adhesive.

A new polythene receptacle sac with tubing attached is suspended by a wire hanger on the bed or wheelchair and the polythene bag and condom connecting tube are joined firmly together. It is a wise precaution to protect the bed with a polythene plastic undersheet.

A leg bag is also available and this is attached to the leg of the patient who is using a wheelchair, by two Velcro straps which are cut to the length of the circumference of the patient's legs.

Regular use of the condom device may cause soreness of the glans penis of the patient. Castelani's Paint (B.P.) is used to cover the sore area and to create a firm surface.

Rehabilitation

The rehabilitation of the patient is the function of a large team who are specialized in the care of the paralysed patients.

The medical staff

In addition to the medical officer directly in charge of the unit in which the patient is nursed, help may be required from consultants who have other special skills; neurology, radiology, orthopaedics, urology, gynaecology, general medicine, general surgery and psychiatry are some of the specialist fields which may be needed for the paralysed patient.

Progression from bed to wheelchair

After the lesion occurs it is inevitable that the patient is nursed horizontally for a long period until there are indications of union and repair at the fracture site. If there are no complications to prevent progress to mobilization this considered by the medical officer of the unit. The site of the fracture may be given a temporary support, such as a sorbo rubber collar or a spinal support, to avoid further trauma at the site of the lesion.

There must be gradual progression to a more upright position from the horizontal posture. As the patient has physiologically adapted the cardio-vascular system to the supine position and the blood vessel walls may be flaccid, due to paralysis, the patient must be given ample time to gain ability to maintain a blood volume in cranial and thoracic cavities as there is a tendency for it to gravitate towards the lower parts of the body. A bed which can be gradually raised at one end to elevate the head to a higher level than the feet may be of use provided it can be made horizontal quickly should the need arise. Once the patient learns to tolerate the upright position in bed a trial movement to wheelchair should be made. At first this is tried with the legs at the same level as the pelvis and then the feet are allowed to rest on the foot supports of the wheelchair.

If there should be distress such as vertigo, weakness or fear, the position of the patient is altered by tilting the chair or raising the legs of the patient. Deep breathing or abdominal palpation may also help. If the problem is persistent and there is no improvement after several days the use of a vasoconstrictor drug, prior to attempting to elevate the patient, may be ordered by the medical officer. It is preferable that the body learns to compensate for the postural change without the aid of the drug however.

Physiotherapy

Efficient rehabilitation of paralysed patients is unlikely without the help of skilled and conscientious physiotherapy staff. They are part of the team who are essential for the intensive care of the patient on his admission and they must work for him right through to his return to his home.

There are so many aspects of physiotherapy care of the paralysed patient that they are best classified in list form:

EARLY
1 Improving breating methods of both tetraplegic and paraplegic patients.
2 Helping the patient to cough and clear the bronchioles of mucus.
3 Maintaining musculature or unparalysed muscles so as to prevent wasting.
4 Preventing contractures of muscles.
5 Preventing stiffness of joints.
6 Inhibiting excessive reflex action.

LATER
  Teaching methods of:
1 Regaining balance(Fig. 5.21 a, b and c).
2 Transferring from bed to chair and chair to bed.
3 Transferring to and from the toilet.
4 Transferring to and from bath or shower.

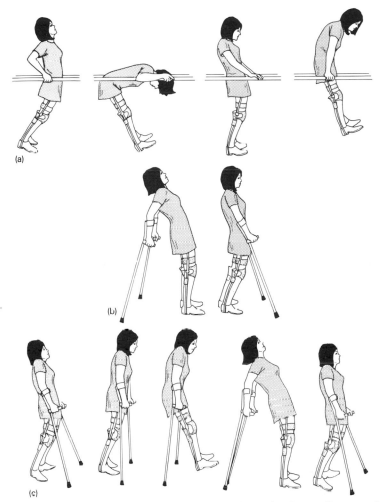

Fig. 5.21. (a) Stretch exercises on parallel bars. (b) Balancing on elbow crutches. (c) Swing through gait.

5 'Press ups'—developing automatic habits in the patient who must elevate his buttocks and sacrum from his wheelchair at frequent intervals using his arms (Fig. 5.16).

6 Standing in calipers or a special walking frame.

7 Mobility—i.e. walking in calipers (only useful for patient with low lesions). (Fig. 5.22).

8 Picking up items from the ground.

9 Wheelchair management.

10 Sports activities—netball, swimming, etc.

11 Strengthening the musculature of the pectoral girdle.

(a)

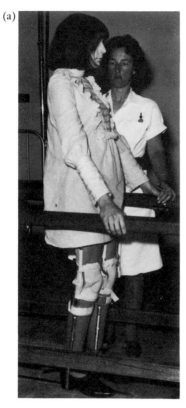

(b)

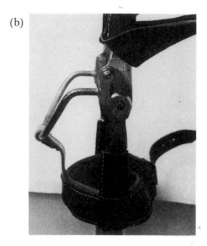

Fig. 5.22. (a) Patient balancing in parallel bars; see also Fig. 5.21(a). (b) The locking device on the knee hinge of a caliper.

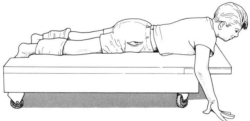

Fig. 5.23. 'Riding the turtle'. This exercise is designed to prevent hip flexion and decubitus ulcers.

12 'Riding the turtle'—an exercise designed to prevent hip flexion and decubitus ulcers.

All these activities are related to the patient's ability to balance himself without the use of the lower limbs. This is a difficult task and one of the prime functions of the physiotherapist is to establish new patterns of balancing so that the patient does not fall over. She requires support from all the other members of the spinal unit team.

Occupational therapy and paraplegia

The spinal injuries patient with paraplegia wil normally be managed in a Spinal Injuries Unit. Within this unit there is a section which is provided for the rehabilitation of the patients as follows:

(a) to return to employment and earning

(b) to using public transport, swing-doors, shops and the other impedimenta which are part of everyday life

(c) to manage his own activities of daily living

(d) to train him in sports activities which can be practised from a wheelchair and will compensate, in a little way for his frustrations

(e) to provide activities which will improve all the musculature which remains for his use

and

(f) to efficiently use wheelchairs.

The unit is staffed by several forms of hospital discipline but the occupational therapy staff usually predominates.

As the paraplegic patient of often a young person who was injured in some activity related to youth, his or her condition reaches a level of stability and with good personal management by the patient he will not deteriorate and will often improve. The approach to the patients activity therefore can usually be dynamic and vigorous. Many acquire skills which they would never have gained without the sequelae of their injury. Much of this related to the optimism engendered in the patient by the staff of the spinal injuries unit as well as the intelligence level and love of living.

The bedfast parplegic

The earliest management by the occupational therapist will occur when the patient is still confined to his bed. Collaborating with the physiotherapy staff the musculature of the trunk, pectoral girdle, neck, arms and hands are all improved in function and their capacity to work raised to a higher level than existed before injury. These muscles will enable the patient to substitute arms for legs in moving from bed to chair, and chair to transport; they are also essential in raising the body from the chair in preventing decubitus ulcers (see page 132). Another occupational therapy need is for the spinal injuries patient with arm and hand involvement in the lesion to develop methods of transferring food from plate or cup to mouth and attending to facial and oral toilet and cosmetic arrangement.

The paraplegic in a wheelchair

Most of the patient's waking life is to be spent in this device; crutch-walking and standing is of limited use. From the moment when the patient moves into a wheelchair for the first time he or she is moving towards independence and this move must be encouraged. The patient must be permitted to do things and training is directed always to self-attainment, and the paraplegic who tends to a lazy approach with a dependence on sympathetic bystanders and family must be suitably dealt with; self-reliance is good for morale.

Working practice

There are many aspects of this and the heading applies to the positioning of wheelchairs, the height of working surfaces and machines, balancing of workshop equipment and much besides. The patient must learn about such matters and apply them in the home, in the bathroom, in the hobbies room, in the office, in the factory, at the drawing board, in the kitchen working surface or in any other area the patient should find him or herself. The practicality of relating the heights of chairs, stools, carseats, cushions, footrests, sinks and washbasins, tabletops, sinks, switches and taps now forms an important part of living and modifications to all equipment the patient uses daily must be made.

Balancing

Paraplegia leads to an understanding of the importance of the lower half of the trunk and legs to sitting and standing (Fig. 5.24 a and b). This ability to balance the patient must re-learn. Applying and removing calipers, rising from the floor to a chair, standing with crutches, sitting with good posture constantly adjusting the centre of gravity by reflex action are essential skills in progression to independence.

Home design

Modifications to a dwelling are essential. There is often a case for building a home especially for a chairbound and paralysed person. If this is not feasible there are many modifications to the standard house which can be made and the occupational therapist may serve as advisor in such matters. Financial aid must be sought and the medical social case-worker can advise on this.

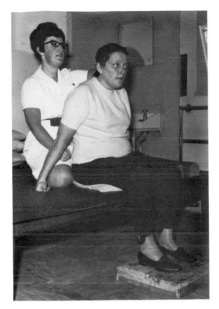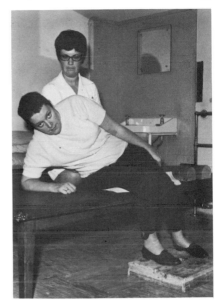

Fig. 5.24.   (a) and (b). Exercises to help the paraplegic patient to regain balance.

Transport

The paraplegic person can drive a modified automobile and there are many forms of modification available for handwriting.

The social caseworker (See also Chapter 13, page 269)

The length of stay of a patient in a spinal injuries unit often depends on the efforts of the social caseworker. She works towards the discharge of the patient to his home and family. In the simplest terms this may mean orientating the family to accepting a chairbound invalid among them. In more complex terms it involves complete rehousing of the patient in a bungalow with ramps instead of stairs or steps, doors wide enough to receive a wheelchair, modified bathroom and toilet facilities, with light switches, door handles and other devices at wheelchair height.

Financially and legally there is much to be done. Money must be found for the patient's family during his holiday stay. He must not become distressed through worrying about their welfare or about debts which are mounting because of his unemployment through hospitalization. Legal advice may be needed to gain the compensation which is due to the patient from the accident and the social caseworker may help in arranging this.

The disablement resettlement officer (see also Chapter 13, page 270).

This worker is the liaison between the hospital, the patient's employer, government retraining centres and a new employer if one must be found. There are many situations in employment which can be found for a chair-bound person of reasonable intelligence.

Transport

A vital factor in helping the paralysed patient to enjoy a full life after rehabilitation in his transport. There are many forms of vehicle available, from conventional cars specially adapted for the disabled to simple electrically-propelled vehicles.

An adequate number of hand-propelled wheelchairs is also necessary, e.g. one light folding transit chair; one for use at home and one for use at work.

6 : Progressive Diseases of the Spinal Cord

Introduction

In addition to acute failure of conduction of impulses in the spinal cord as already outined, due to injury, infection or sudden cessation of the blood supply, there are a considerable number of chronic progressive spinal cord disorders. Some of these are due to chronic infection, others to progressive impairment of the blood supply to to slowly growing tumours, others to a biochemical deficiency which may be extrinsic or intrinsic (often termed biogenesis). Tumours may be extradural or intradural; intradural tumours are divided into intra- and extramedullary. The tumours themselves may be simple or malignant, and malignant tumours may be primary or secondary. There are, in addition, a number of ill-understood progresive disorders of the spinal cord, some of which appear to have a hereditary basis and whose onset is often in childhood or adolescence, such as Friedreich's ataxia. Others, such as motor neurone disease or lateral sclerosis, occur during the latter half of life of some, such as multiple sclerosis may occur at any age. In other cases, such as in subacute combined degeneration of the spinal cord, it is known that this is due to a specific chemical deficiency and is frequently associated with pernicious anaemia or a folic acid deficiency. In all of these conditions the mode of onset is slow and insidious. In addition to impairment of muscle control leading to spastic paraplegia, similar to that seen in other upper motor neurone disorders, there may be varying types of paralysis, loss of sensation, pain and loss of sphincter control. While the specific treatment of a spinal cord disorder is primarily a matter for the neurologist or neurosurgeon, the alleviation of the results of a chronic disease of the spinal cord largely falls on the physiotherapist, occupational therapist and orthopaedic surgeon. The control of muscular spasm, the prevention and correction of deformity and the provision of various aids are all very important factors in making life tolerable for the unfortunate victim of chronic progressive spinal paralysis. In essence, the measures are similar to those which are used for patients with acute paraplegia though, of course, they must be modified according to the amount of neurological function is retained.

Chapter 6

Relevant applied anatomy and physiology

The control of most activities in the body is by the central nervous system; a general title for the brain and spinal cord. This is composed entirely of delicate nervous tissue and supporting connective tissue and blood vessels; without protection the central nervous system would be vulnerable to injury. It is, therefore, entirely surrounded by bone in the form of the cranium and vertebral column. Inside the cavity which encloses the central nervous system, i.e. the cranial cavity and neural canal, is a protective membrane called the theca.

The terms upper motor neurone lesion and lower motor neurone lesion will be used in this chapter. It is now necessary to define these terms.

Upper motor neurones

Refer to Fig. 6.1 as you read this section. The so-called upper motor neurones in the central nervous system have the main function of trans-

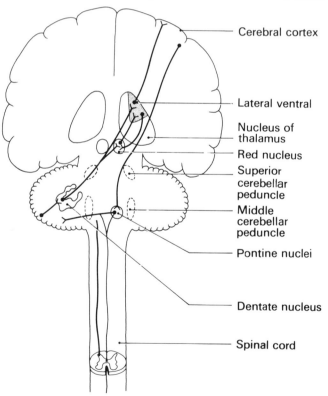

Cerebral cortex

Lateral ventral

Nucleus of thalamus

Red nucleus

Superior cerebellar peduncle

Middle cerebellar peduncle

Pontine nuclei

Dentate nucleus

Spinal cord

Fig. 6.1. The upper motor neurones.

ferring the impulses, which arise on the cortex or surface of the cerebrum, to other parts of the central nervous system. They form nervous tracts or pathways along which the impulses pass. Thus there are pathways between the cerebrum and cerebellum; others between the cerebellum and mid-brain and medulla oblongata; there are also pathways from the brain stem down the spinal cord and in the reverse direction. Every part of the healthy central nervous system has a communication via such pathways with other parts of the brain and spinal cord; these pathways are normally clear and free of obstruction.

Any pathological condition which impedes the passage of nervous impulses along these pathways between the cortex of the brain and the relevant segment of the spinal cord is known as an upper motor neurone lesion.

Lesions of upper motor neurones

In the case of upper motor neurone lesions many different varities of impairment of upper motor neurone control can occur. For instance, disorders of the spinal cord may, if they affect the posterior roots or columns (as in tabes dorsalis) as well as the upper motor neurones give rise to loss of reflexes, diminution of muscle tone and disorder of joints known as neuropathic joints (Fig. 6.3.). At a slightly higher level, interruption of all upper motor neurones as, for example, in traumatic paraplegia or certain spinal tumours, will give rise to increased muscle tone, exaggeration of the flexor reflexes, diminution of the extensor reflexes which are inhibited, and a characteristic posture. Flexed and adducted hips, flexed knees and equinus deformity of the feet may develop if the condition is not treated.

Other diseases of the spinal cord such as Friedreich's ataxia, disseminated sclerosis, and syringomyelia may give rise to similar disorders.

At a higher level, disorders of the brain stem and cerebellum may give

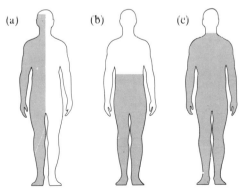

Fig. 6.2. Types of paralysis. (a) Hemiplegia; (b) paraplegia; (c) tetraplegia.

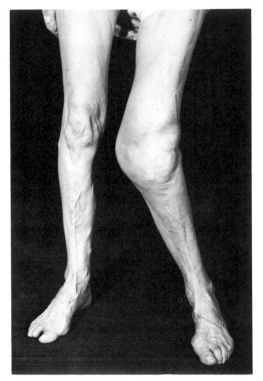

Fig. 6.3.   A neuropathic joint.

rise to disorders of posture, spontaneous increased rigidity, and spontaneous fine rhythmical tremor as in Parkinson's disease, intentional tremor as in diseases of the cerebellum due either to a tumour or to disseminated sclerosis, or spontaneous writhing movements—athetosis.

At a still higher level, lesions of the motor cortex of the cerebellum may give rise to complete loss of voluntary movement or partial weakness and the increased loss of muscle tone. According to the extent of the paralysis it is classified as:

Monoplegia: one limb. Hemiplegia: the arm and leg on the same side.
Paraplegia: both legs. Tetraplegia: all four limbs.

According to the exact situation of the lesion the limbs may be spastic ataxic or hypertonic, or there may be spontaneous movements, e.g. athetoid.

Lower motor neurones

Refer to Fig. 6.4 as you read this section. As the central nervous system is protected within its bony cavity, there must be a connecting nervous tract or pathway between the spinal cord and all of the bodily structures which

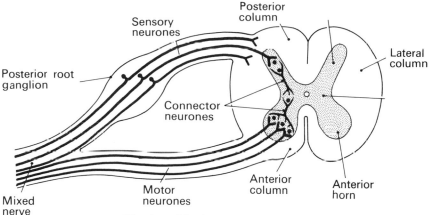

Fig. 6.4. The lower motor neurones.

are external to the theca. This communicating pathway is usually a spinal nerve which may also be called a peripheral nerve (see Chapter 3).

The spinal nerve arises from one side of a segment of the spinal cord by two roots which join before passing out of the neural canal to that part of the body which it supplies. Any pathological condition which damages, breaks or obstructs the nervous pathway (from its origin within the spinal cord segment along the spinal nerve to its destination, a peripheral organ such as muscles) is referred to as a lower motor neurone lesion.

Lesions of lower motor neurones

The causes of lower motor neurone lesions include anterior poliomyelitis and other virus infections, peripheral nerve lesions   traumatic, toxic and infective, e.g. leprosy—and diseases of the motor endplate and muscle.

It is fairly easy to understand that if, for instance, the muscles which dorsiflex the foot are paralysed, the normally acting plantar flexors are liable to produce a fixed equinus deformity.

The treatment of lower motor neurone lesions—that is if the lesion itself is untreatable—is to prevent deformity arising by suitable splints and exercises. If deformity arises, correction is by lengthening the tendons of contracted muscles and preventing recurrence of the deformity for example, by tendon transplant. If the anterior tibial muscles are paralysed, the tibialis posterior muscle is transferred through the interosseous membrane to the dorsum of the foot. In certain circumstances fusion operations to fix or arthrodese flail joints are necessary.

All skeletal muscle are innervated by a peripheral motor nerve arising from the anterior horn cell and supplying a number of muscle fibres; the whole is known as the lower motor neurone complex. The exact control of the muscles of the limbs and trunk in standing and moving is a complex procedure based on what is known as the stretch reflex, i.e. the reflex contraction of muscle fibres when the muscle is stretched. The stretch reflex itself is subjected to a complex of fibres known as upper motor neurone fibres originating in the brain.

Disorders of muscle action and muscle imbalance are divided into two main types: upper motor neurone lesions and lower motor neurone lesions. Muscle imbalance leads to deformed posture, abnormal gait, abnormal movements and ultimately to fixed deformities.

From the surgeon's point of view the essential aim is avoid the development of fixed deformities and, in particular, pathological dislocation due to unequal muscle pull. A careful assessment must be made, therefore, of all muscles which are too active; these can be balanced either by tenotomy, myotomy, neurectomy or muscle transfer. Upper limb function is dependent on good voluntary control and good tactile postural sensation. Upper motor neurone lesions may cause poor control of movements or coarse or fine tremor. In addition, in all diseases of the brain they may be a varying degree of mental impairment, deafness, impairment of sight or eye control, difficulty in coordinating swallowing and breathing, or in articulating.

Comparison of the effects of neurone lesions

Upper motor neurone lesions
1   Spastic paralysis of the affected limbs. 2   Little or no muscle wasting.
3   Exaggerated reflexes. 4   Local temperature and colour changes absent; generalized effects on the skin may be present. 5   Babinski's sign positive.
6   Absent abdominal responses.

Lower motor neorone lesions.
1   Flaccid paralysis of the affected limbs. 2   Severe wasting of muscles.
3   Absence of reflexes. 4   Local temperature and colour changes; of the skin of the affected part. 5   Babinski's sign negative or no response. 6   Reduced tone

TABES DORSALIS
Nowadays this condition is rare. It is characterized by ataxia, loss of joint sense, hypotonicity and areflexia. It may lead to the important complication of a swollen flail joint (neuropathic arthropathy or Charcot joint). Such a joint requires external support—e.g. by a caliper. Occasionally fixation (arthrodesis) is used, but this is not normally advisable. Although pain

appreciation from external stimulation is deficient, spontaneous (so-called lightning) pains may occur.

FRIEDREICH'S ATAXIA

Like disseminated sclerosis, this may affect the cerebellum and the spinal cord. It develops in childhood, is progressive and may cause severe deformities, especially of the spine. The prognosis for life is poor as the heart muscle is usually weak.

Occasionally treatment of the scoliotic spine may be necessary, either by external or internal supports, to enable the child to sit upright.

SYRINGOMYELIA

This is a slowly progressive disorder of the spinal cord which affects

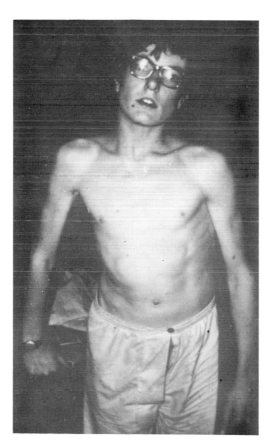

Fig. 6.5. (a) Syringomyelia. Frontal view.

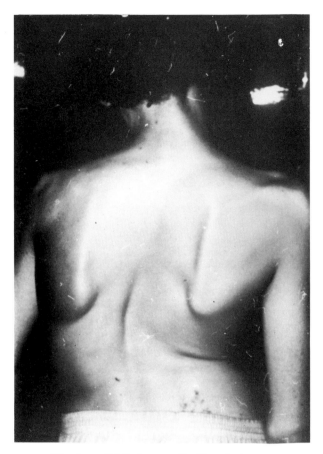

Fig. 6.5. (b) Syringomyelia. Dorsal view.

young adults. It may lead to spasticity of the legs, scoliosis, wasting of the small hand muscles, neuropathic joints and trophic lesions of the skin.

Orthopaedic measures may be required for the spinal deformity and for the spastic legs.

DISSEMINATED SCLEROSIS

This condition may manifest itself in several ways. In the cerebellar form there will be ataxia, incoordination of movement, intention tremor, dysarthria, and nystagmus. Specific orthopaedic treatment does not help cerebellar lesions, though measures such as Frankel's exercises and walking in front of a mirror may give the patient confidence.

In the spinal form with spasticity, measures to prevent or correct deformity and reduce excessive muscle tone as for cerebral palsy may help the patient. Occasionally, supporting splints—e.g. below-knee irons—help a patient to walk. The disease runs a chronic intermittent fluctuating course, and every effort should be made to keep the patient ambulant. Ultimately, impairment of sphincter control is likely to occur and add to the patient's miseries.

The management of patients with chronic affections of the spinal cord

Recent progress in neurology and neurosurgery offers much help to the patient with disorders of the brain and spinal cord, as there are many advances in drug therapy and surgery. Nevertheless, these patients must often modify their way of life so as to adjust to their permanent residual disability. They come from a whole range of age groups, but those who require most help from nursing and physiotherapy staff may be classified as:

1 the very young who have a congenital condition.
2 any young adults who suffer from progressive neurological disorders.
3 elderly adults usually with cerebrovascular disorders.

All groups present different management problems.

Emotional and psychological management

Patients who develop chronic regressive conditions of the central nervous system present problems of communication to the medical officer who is caring for them. What should one tell the patient? How much is it good for the patient to know? How much do the relatives wish the patient to know? Do the realtives want to maintain a façade which prevents the patient knowing that he is suffering from a chronic neurological disorder which will not improve and will steadily get worse?

The method of transmission to the patient of the knowledge of the condition, from which he is suffering depends upon several factors:

(a) The depth of the patient's knowledge of medical matters. Obviously a doctor, nurse or physiotherapist patient who is able to recognize the symptoms and signs must be given all the information required.

(b) The intelligence of the patient is related to his desire to know. Some patients, for their own peace of mind maintain their own façade behind which they hide and pretend that all is well. They do not wish to know about their condition.

(c) The emotional response of the patient. Some are stoical but others may tend to become hysterical.

Most patients with multiple sclerosis are dismayed and despondent although they cloak this with stoicism; a minority show a cheerfulness which is euphoric.

The doctor in charge of the patient will assess all factors in deciding how much and what to tell the patient. There is no doubt that all information about the condition should be given to the patient in small amounts at a time over a long period of days, weeks or months. Too detailed an account of the pathology in too large a quantity, at one time can only cause shock and severe depression.

The management problems

The patients who have multiple sclerosis present a variety of different symptoms and signs.

Remissions and relapses

There are periods when the symptoms appear to improve and others when they get worse. The improvements tend to cause elation and the regression cause depression.

In either case the patient needs much encouragement and support. Talking to friends, relations, and nursing, medical and physiotherapy staff can do much to help.

Paralysis and paresis of a limb or limbs

The patient develops clumsiness of movement at an early stage of his condition and this may be his first reason for calling in the doctor. The paralysis may affect one or both lower limbs in which case gait and walking will be disordered and as this regresses the patient will be unable to walk without support from hand rails, or sticks or crutches; eventually he or she will be unable to move except in a wheelchair. Falls may occur so that facial bruising and cuts or more serious injury are common events.

The nursing and physiotherapy management of this problem is mainly to assist the patient to maintain his personal independence for as long as he can. Progressions to various aids to locomotion will be necessary; thus one stick, then two sticks, elbow crutches, then quadripods, and eventually wheelchairs will be necessary.

Paraesthesia, numbness and loss of sensation

This results from involvement of the sensory fibres of the posterior columns of the spinal cord. The patient's awareness of the position of his limbs is lost and he is unaware of the position of his limbs without looking at them. Even when he sees them he may have problems in 'accepting' that a limb is his because he cannot feel it. This results in an 'ataxic' gait as he staggers because he cannot 'plant' his feet where they should be.

An additional problem is his loss of skin sensation and the possibility of damage because of burning or excoriation due to friction. He must be aware of the need to protect his skin from hazards. Hot radiators and pipes, electric fires and bed–heating devices must be guarded; straps and clips on clothing or darns on socks or tight footwear may cause skin lesions and must be avoided.

Dysarthria (slurred speech)

This is a common problem and one which can be very frustrating for the patient. The difficulties which this problem creates are many. Normal conversation and communion with the family is lost. Requests may be misunderstood. The use of the telephone is often denied the patient: The listener may be intolerant of the inarticulate patient and refuse him the time needed to communicate.

Speech therapy has a place but the main need of the patient is time to talk slowly and repeat any misunderstood phrases. The speech also improves on occasion but then regresses. Eventually normal communication is lost and sign or reading communication is all that is possible.

Bladder dysfunction

This may take several forms:

1 *Precipitancy of micturition:* The patient is aware of the need to pass urine from a full bladder but cannot retain the urine long enough to reach the lavatory and the whole bladder content is voided into clothing.

2 *Retention of urine:* The bladder is full, the patient is aware of this (and may even be in pain) but the urethral sphincter is in spasm and the urine cannot be expelled. Eventually the urine is forced through in a dribble. This is known as retention with overflow.

3 *Incontinence of urine:* In this case the patient is unable to retain the urine in the baldder. This may be because of a paralysed urethral sphincter. The urine is passed out as soon as it reaches the bladder from the ureters.

The management of the patient's urinary problems depends upon the individual's needs.

THE FEMALE PATIENT

Management of the incontinent female patient (with any clinical condition) is always a problem. The opening of the urethra in the folds of the vulva, the absence of any means of attaching a collecting device to the opening and the position of the vulva under the trunk when seated creates problems which many experts have tried without success to resolve. Probably the UROVAC developed at the National Rehabilitation Centre, Dublin, is the most effective. (Fig. 6.6).

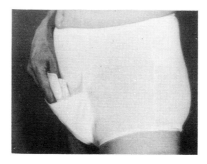

Fig. 6.6.   A urine collecting device for use on a female patient.

Catheterization

The presence of an indwelling catheter, which must be retained *in situ* constantly, can and will result in infection usually of a chronic low-grade nature. This causes the deterioration of the general health of the patient and would require a repeated or prolonged antibiotic regime which is undesirable. Silastic catheters have been found to be less irritant to the mucose of the urethra but infection must supervene eventually.

It is preferable to avoid catheterization and modern attitudes to urinary management consider that catherization of any patient is rarely necessary.

Surgical intervention

A surgical procedure may be performed to create an 'ileal loop' bladder. (See Fig. 6.7). The ureters of the patient are connected to an isolated segment of intestine which opens on to the anterior abdominal wall into a collecting bag which is attached by adhesive to surround the stoma which protrudes.

Such surgical procedures may not be considered appropriate in disseminated sclerosis patients because of the complexity of the paralysis. The problem which is relieved may be replaced by another which is more troublesome.

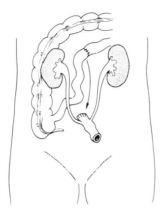

Fig. 6.7.   An ileal loop bladder (see also Fig. 5.20).

Incontinence clothing

The use of waterproof pants with absorbant pads inserted to soak up the excreted urine may be the only feasible method of managing most female patients with the problem of constant dribble of small quantities of urine. These can only be satisfactory if the pads are regularly replaced at intervals. In all methods of managing the problems of the incontinent patient the standards of personal hygiene must be high. When incontinence pads are in use the daily or twice daily bath is essential both for the patient and her attendants and family.

THE MALE PATIENT

The structure of the male genitalia is more suited to the efficient use of incontinence devices. The condom device, if properly fitted and used, is probably the most effective. The use of this is described in Chapter 5 on page 138. The merit of its use is that no interval interference with the bladder, as would be needed in catherization, is necessary.

If the condom device is properly connected to Urisac bags, for either day or night use, the patient can remain clean, dry and comfortable. Again, a daily bath and regular shaving of the pubic hair ensures the self-esteem of the patient.

Visual disturbance

Diplopia (double vision), blurring of vision, temporary blindness of an eye and inability to focus both eyes on, for example, a line of print may occur. The ophthalmologist may help with some aspects of this problem but it is often one to be accepted. When one of the few pleasures remaining for the patient may be reading or watching television, loss of visual efficiency is a severe blow.

Miscellaneous problems

These are less common but nevertheless irksome to the patient:

Vertigo: A feeling of dizziness and 'everything whirling around' because of interference with the patient's balance mechanism.

Deafness: This occurs when the auditory area of the brain has been affected.

Dysphagia: Difficulty in swallowing food and drink.

Trigeminal neuralgia: This is severe paroxysmal pain in the side of the face when the relevant area of the brain is affected.

Epilepsy: The patient has fits. These can often be controlled with the specific drugs for epilepsy.

Adaptation of the patient's home

Given full financial support, expert advice and a suitable house much can be done to improve the lot of a patient with a chronic spinal lesion. Probably the best type of dwelling for adaptation is a spacious bungalow cited on a level plane and without steps and slopes. If the home is purpose-built it can be entirely related to the needs of the patient with doorways, ramps for wheelchairs, bathroom fitting, light switches and power points and other fittings designed to meet the needs of the patient in a wheelchair who must live within a limiting regime. The following are considerations in designing or adapting a home for a patient with a chronic affection of the spinal cord:

1   *Structure for building:* As stated, the building should preferably be on one level and spacious. All doorways should be wide enough for a wheelchair to pass easily through and door handles at the height the patient can reach them. There should be accommodation such as a bathroom and bedroom so that a separate suite can be provided, if necessary, for the patient.

2 *Heating:* The process of dressing may be long and tedious for the patient. The morning toilet may take up to ninety minutes or more and if the patient is also cold he will become doubly exhausted in the process. Double-glazing, heat insulation and an effective central heating system are necessary.

3 *Lighting:* The electrical fittings deserve special consideration. Switches should be lowered and power points raised to enable the patient to operate them by himself. Extra lights may assist the patient in such activities as toilet and reading. Switches which give control of lights and appliances at several points are an advantage.

4 *Coat Hangers, taps, sinks, mirrors, cookers:* (Fig. 6.8). These should all be adapted or adaptable to the patient's needs.

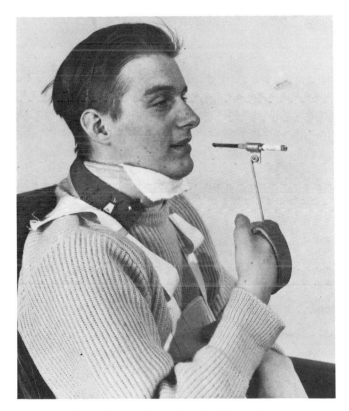

Fig. 6.8. A device for a disabled patient.

5 *Leaning posts:* (Fig. 6.9). The patient putting on trousers, briefs, socks or stockings needs to raise a leg while standing. If the patient can stand,

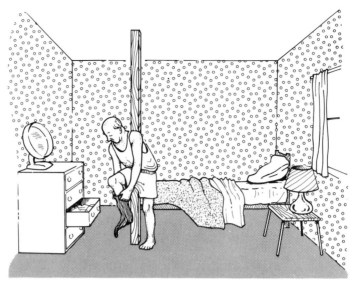

Fig. 6.9. A leaning post to assist a paralysed patient to dress himself.

even badly, he will stand even better by leaning against an upright strong post attached to floor and ceiling.

6   *Access to lawn or garden:* (Fig. 6.10). A double door from the patient's suite to the garden is a joy.

7   *Extra garage facilities:* Motorized invalid transport and wheelchairs require storage. Many of these facilities are expensive accessories which

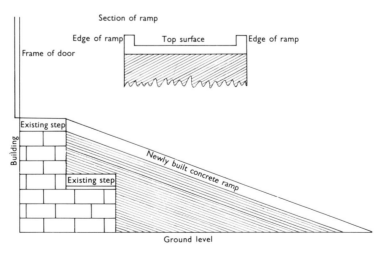

Fig. 6.10. A ramp down from a house to allow easier wheelchair axis.

are beyond the means of many people. However, the social services of many countries and philanthropic institutions may have the legislation or finance to supply these facilities.

General attitudes

The patient with a chronic spinal lesion has a poor prognosis although many live to enjoy a long if limited life. It is essential to maintain a high standard of grooming, personal hygiene and cosmetic care and pressure from relatives and attendants may be needed to encourage a depressed or apathetic patient to keep up appearances. Full dressing should always be encouraged and a slovenly 'dressing gown and slippers' attitude discouraged.

An alternating regime of rest and activity is probably best. When the patient is able, full activity at work or hobby should be carried out. If the patient is tired he should rest. Prolonged futile inactivity, sitting still and staring into the distance or dozing are not good and contribute to joint stiffness and muscle wasting. The patient should be trained to sit well, in a chair most suited to his height and size.

Stimulation by communication with people outside the usual orbit is essential. Memberships of clubs or community or church groups is good for morale.

Feeding should be ample but must not contribute to obesity. A balanced diet of a quantity to meet the calorific needs of the patient in the light of his limited activity should be given. Excessive carbohydrate intake must be avoided.

Ultimately the patient will become fully dependent. Consideration must then be given to the most suitable premises for the management of the patient. If there is only one person attempting to give full care to the patient there is a danger that the health of the attendant may suffer. Then there is a case for moving the patient into a suitable institution where adequate staff and facilities exist for the proper care of the patient.

7 : Acute Head Injuries

Relevant anatomy and physiology

The cranium is a hard box which contains and protects the delicate nervous tissue forming the brain. Within the box the hemispheres of the cerebrum are supported, at their posterior lobes, on a transverse sling of membrane derived from the duramater. To allow the spinal cord to connect with the mid-brain, the tentorium cerebelli as the transverse sling is called, is penetrated. The junction of the mid-brain and spinal cord is in direct relationship to this opening in the tentorium.

In acceleration or deceleration incidents when the skull and its contents are jerked suddenly either backwards or forwards the tentorial sling acts in much the same way as a guillotine and the mid-brain may be severely damaged (Fig. 7.1). Such an injury results in unconsciousness which may only last a short time in a mild lesion or a long time in a severe lesion.

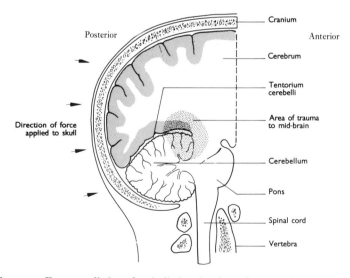

Fig. 7.1. Force applied to the skull showing how the tentorium cerebelli may injure the brain.

In addition there will probably be severe bruising or even tearing of the lobes of the brain from which there is limited recovery or no recovery. If the parietal lobes are involved there will be paralysis because the motor areas of the brain, which control the movement of the limbs, are affected. As the motor area of one of the parietal lobes influences the opposite side of the body in a left-sided hemiplegia and vice versa. If the cerebellum is the site of the lesion there will be unsteadiness and loss of coordination of muscle function.

Recovery from any damage to nervous tissue, such as that forming the brain, is slow. The patient may suffer the effects of the injury for months or years. The process of recovery cannot be hurried but wise management can assist recovery and unwise measures delay recovery.

The first aid management of the patient with head injuries

1 The conscious patient

Although a patient who has received a blow on the head or has a head wound may be conscious and cooperative, it must not be assumed that all is well and that no further action is necessary. If there is any bleeding occurring within the cranial cavity the brain will be under pressure which will increase and result in the later deterioration of the patient who may not be under observation at that time. It is always wise to ensure that anybody who has had a severe blow on the head, with or without amnesia or transient unconsciousness, is examined by a doctor and is kept under efficient observation for a twenty-four hour period after the injury.

2 The unconscious patient

In a first-aid situation it is unlikely that the cause of the unconsciousness can be diagnosed with certainty and there are many causes of loss of consciousness. For instance, the combination of alcohol or other drugs and a bruised head may present a difficult problem in a differential diagnosis. Diabetes, epilepsy and other medical conditions must also be considered. Once any obvious factor, which would result in further deterioration before a patient reaches hospital, has been dealt with the main efforts must be:
1 maintenance of an adequate airflow into and out of the patient's lungs.
2 prevention of inhalation of anything which would obstruct the airway.
3 arrest of bleeding from wounds.
4 protection of the patient from the elements.

5 transportation to the most suitable centre available for the management
of a head injuries patient.

The unconscious patient is in danger of death because he may be unable
to breath. The prime function of anyone rendering first aid is to clear any
obstruction to the respiratory passages. The indication, to the observer,
that the patient is having respiratory problems is that the patient is making
violent respiratory efforts against the obstruction. The shoulders and thorax
jerk violently, the face and eyes are engorged and discoloured.

The obstruction may be the flaccid tongue which has fallen back into
the pharynx as the patient faces upwards (Fig. 7.2). This is dealt with by
altering the position of the patient to the semiprone (Fig. 7.3). In this
position the tongue and debris tend to fall forwards and out of the mouth.

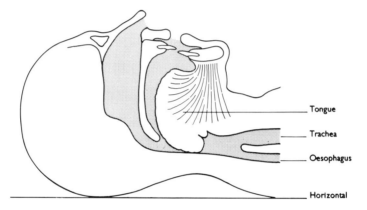

Fig. 7.2.   An obstructed pharynx caused by the tongue falling backwards in the
throat of a patient.

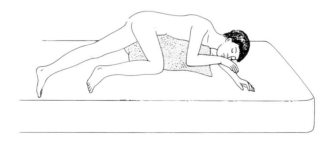

Fig. 7.3.   The position for an unconscious patient.

This position should be the standard 'unconscious patient' position for the
first aid worker to practice. If the mouth and throat are examined by sight
or with fingers it may be that dentures, blood-clots or vomited food are

obstructing and must be removed. If these have already been inhaled, rapid transportation to a hospital where suction apparatus is available, is the most urgent measure to be taken. When breathing has ceased mouth-to-mouth respiration or the use of a resuscitator which insufflates the lungs must be commenced. Oxygen administration is of value only if the airway has been cleared.

Pathology of head injuries

The degree of brain damage in a head injury varies from transient impairment of consciousness (whose micropathology is still largely an enigma) to gross lacerations and destruction of brain tissue leading to severe permanent sequelae. In addition, head injuries may be associated with facial and jaw injuries, damage to eyes and ears and damage to the cervical spine as well as damage to the trunk and limbs in 'high velocity' injuries such as falls from a height or road traffic accidents.

If there has been damage to the dura mater and skull, a cerebrospinal fluid fistula may develop leading to rhinorrhoea or otorrhoea. Such a fistula may lead to infection and meningitis or a brain abscess. Equally, if there is an open fracture of the skull there is a risk of infection of the brain and mininges.

Apart from infection the pathology of brain injuries may conveniently be divided into early and late changes.

Early changes include oedema, contusions, lacerations, vascular occlusion, haemorrhage—intracerebral, extracerebral, intradural and extradural —as well as direct traumatic destruction of brain cells.

Late manifestations include gliosis (intracerebral scarring), vascular occlusion, infection, dural adhesions, subdural haematoma, internal hydrocephalus and cerebrospinal fistula.

It is hardly necessary to point out that loss of consciousness associated with a fall or bruising or laceration of the scalp, does not necessarily mean that the loss of consciousness is due to the head injury. The patient might have lost consciousness for a 'medical' reason such as epilepsy, cerebrovascular accident (including a cerebral aneurysm), hypoglycaemia, uraemia, drug intoxication, etc. and then fallen and struck his head.

From the practical point of view, the most important pathological condition which should be excluded in the early stages is progressive extradural haemorrhage. Diffuse intracerebral haemorrhage cannot usually be successfully treated by direct surgical intervention. Although avoiding anaemia and venous congestion may improve the prognosis, restoring adequate oxygenation is the first consideration in any head injury.

In addition to controlling haemorrhage, penetrating wounds require the appropriate wound toilet and suitable measures to avoid intracranial infection. At a later stage, surgical intervention may also be required to repair cerebrospinal fluid fistulae, remove indriven spicules of bones, a subdural cyst or area of gliosis or to control a leaking aneurysm of the circle.

Clinical examination

Repeated clinical examination of an unconscious patient is most important and is the safest way of avoiding the tragedy of failing to diagnose potentially curable lesions.

In addition, to noting carefully any signs of external damage, it is often desirable to shave the head to facilitate examination. The patient must be examined for signs of injuries elsewhere—particularly the eyes, ears, jaws, nasopharynx, chest, neck and abdomen.

Neurological examination will include the estimation of the depth of unconsciousness, the state of the pupils and their reactions, the tone of the limb muscles and the blood pressure, pulse and respiration rates.

Levels of unconsciousness

Levels of unconsciousness can conveniently be divided into:
1   light, i.e. can be roused and answers to simple questions.
2   responds to light stimuli and obeys simple commands.
3   responds to strong stimuli—e.g. bright light, pinching, pinprick but is uncooperative.
4   unconscious but restless.
5   deeply comatose with slowing of heart and respiration rate and increasing pulse pressure.

The total treatment of head injuries is beyond the scope of this book, but above all, anoxia and cyanosis must be relieved—if necessary, by a tracheostomy and artificial respiration. If unconsciousness is prolonged, feeding by an intragastric tube or parenterally, may be necessary, and avoiding pressure sores and limb contractures and care of the bladder will require similar attention as in paraplegia.

The late result of head injuries

As a late result of a head injury, the patient may be left with a varying degree of spastic paralysis—hemiplegia or tetraplegia and the long-term treatment of this is the same as for hemiplegia or tetraplegia resulting from other causes. It should, however, be remembered that residual paralysis is relatively uncommon compared with cerebral symptoms, headaches, dizziness, inability to concentrate, forgetfulness, depression, lack of initiative, irritability, personality changes, etc. It is often difficult to be sure how far such symptoms have an organic basis, i.e. are due to psychological reaction to the accident, particularly if this is the subject of a medico-legal claim. It is surprising if a severe injury which causes prolonged unconsciousness and lengthy retrograde amnesia does not produce permanent organic changes. Equally, it is unlikely that a minor injury, by itself producing only transient impairment of consciousness, will produce permanent changes unless there are pre-existing changes in the brain or its arteries.

EXTRADURAL HAEMORRHAGE (Fig. 7.4)

Although this syndrome is relatively rare, it requires special mention, because to fail to diagnose it is a tragedy. Classically, the patient sustains a head injury, is unconscious for a short period, then apparently recovers completely, but a few hours later, he again becomes unconscious, with a fixed dilated pupil. The treatment is to evacuate the blood clot and stop the bleeding which often comes from the middle meningeal cells. If untreated, the condition is usually fatal. Therefore, if there are reasonable clinical grounds for suspecting the diagnosis, it is often wiser to make burr holes in the skull, rather than wait for the results of sophisticated investigations such as angiography. If treated in time, the prognosis is good in children, but becomes progressively worse with age.

Late sequelae of a head injury may be classified into those for which there is a definite pathological basis with clear-cut physical signs, and those

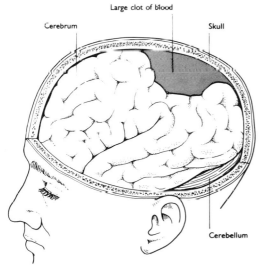

Large clot of blood

Cerebrum   Skull

Cerebellum

Fig. 7.4. Extra-dural haemorrhage compressing the brain.

vague symptoms for which the exact basis is unknown. The latter includes headache; giddiness, inability to concentrate, irritability and personality changes. The true basic causes for such symptoms are largely unknown.

By contrast, there are other well-defined sequelae, including epilepsy, in which an area of gliosis can frequently be demonstrated, and mental impairment and somnolence, often associated with characteristic pupil changes and sometimes hemiparesis which characterize a chronic subdural haematoma.

This last condition, though relatively rare, must always be kept in mind, as onset of symptoms is insidious and unwise lumbar puncture may precipitate fatal medullary coming with respiratory paralysis. If untreated, the condition leads to progressive brain damage, but if treated early by surgical evacuation, the prognosis is good.

THE NURSING MANAGEMENT OF THE PATIENT WITH HEAD INJURIES

Care during prolonged unconsciousness

The patient in an unconscious state is entirely dependent on the nursing and medical staff for survival, hence nursing care must be concentrated and continuous.

This kind of patient is, preferably, nursed in a special unit or cubicle. The position of such patients is altered every two hours as a set routine. The object of changing the patient's position regularly is to prevent decubitus ulcers, to prevent stasis in the renal system and lungs, and to improve circulation in the tissues, and ventilation in the lungs. Thus, the patient is turned from the right lateral position to the recumbent position, then to the left lateral position, at regular recorded intervals.

The clothing and bedding must be light in weight and allow access to the patient's body. Patients in whom the heat-regulating centre of the brain has been damaged may suffer from an excessive rise in temperature, which the nurses will have to reduce by means of electric fans and tepid sponging; they are best nursed without clothing and with their skin exposed to the atmosphere.

Observation

Any unconscious patient's life depends upon good nursing, observation and recording. A process of continual observation is necessary from the moment of admission and it must be a continual uninterrupted process. A half-hourly recording of the observations must be made, and all the nursing staff should be familiar with a standardized form of the observations so that each new nurse coming on duty is aware of the state of the patient and can note changes.

The observation shart (Fig. 7.5) should record in simple clear fashion:

1 *Comments on the level of consciousness*

It is necessary for the nurse to test the patient's level of consciousness by such methods as calling his name, pinching him gently, and examining his eyes to note the pupil's responses to light. Restlessness or confusion must be recorded. As much information as possible should be noted.

Probably the most important record in head injury patients is the level of consciousness, closely followed by the state of the pupils of the eyes; any increase or decrease in size should be recorded; the most significant change would be irregularity of the pupil size.

2 *Pulse rate and blood pressure*

This is a useful guide to changes in the patient's condition. A lowering of the pulse rate and blood pressure would indicate a rise in intracranial pressure and deterioration, requiring surgical intervention in a head injury. Any change must be instantly reported to the doctor in charge.

3 Respiration rate

4 Temperature

5 Fluid balance

Changes in the patient can be rapid and dramatic; instant reporting of such changes is essential.

Patient hygiene

Although the patient is completely unconscious, a good standard of personal hygiene is necessary for survival. A daily bed bath, good oral hygiene and hair care are routine; soiling of the skin is inevitable from bowel and bladder evacuation, hence frequent washing of the genital and and anal area is necessary.

Faecal excretion

Bowel evacuation at regular intervals is necessary. The diet of the patient cannot contain roughage to fill the colon, nevertheless faeces will form and must be removed. Bowel evacuation is a reflex process that is

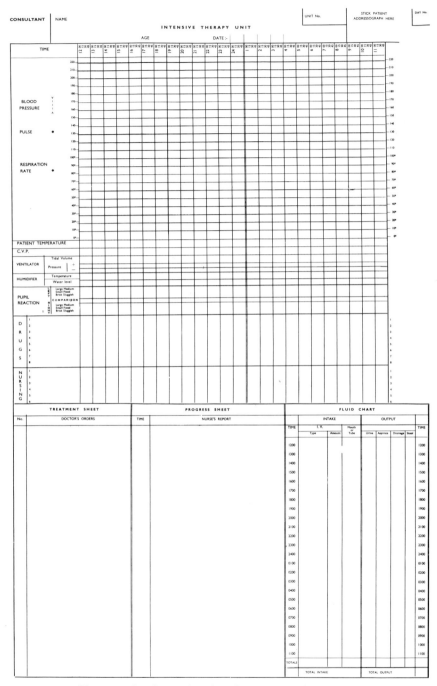

Fig. 7.5. An observation chart for an unconscious patient.

inhibited in the conscious state until it is convenient to evacuate; many an unconscious patient, with no paralysis of the abdomen, will probably return to the primitive reflex state of the infant and defaecate at daily or two-daily intervals depending on diet and previous habits; it is a matter of supplying the receptacle when the patient starts to bear down. In such patients the assistance of enemata or suppositories is not required.

Other unconscious patients, however, become constipated without some stimulation to bowel evacuation. This stimulation consists of the insertion of glycerine or senna suppositories into the rectum, or the use of concentrated enemas commercially available; the use of enemas, consisting of large quantities of fluid, is not recommended as small quantities of faecally-stained fluid tend to ooze long after the initial procedure has been performed. A single semi-solid evacuation is the aim of treatment.

All the body processes in the unconscious patient must be accurately charted, and the fluid intake and output chart, together with the general condition of the patient, will indicate the adequacy of fluid exchange. Intragastric feeding of the patient will be established so that plenty of fluid can be given. A healthy moist appearance to the mucous membranes, a good elasticity or 'tone' to the tissues, and an ample urine output, indicate that the patient is not dehydrated.

Urine excretion

The ability of the patient to pass urine is related to the level of unconsciousness and the return to the primitive reflex bladder emptying of the infant. If the patient can be stimulated to pass urine at regular intervals by sound or sensory skin stimuli, this is preferable to interference by catheterzation. If bladder function is not impaired, the bladder will fill with urine and, when the walls of the bladder are stretched, they will contract downwards. Observation and timing by the nursing staff will let them know when a quantity of urine is present in the bladder. By calling to the patient in some cases, or by application of pressure or cold or warmth to the pubic area, in others, micturition may begin. A condom drainage and urine sac (see Chapter 5, page oo) may be applied to male patients from the commencement of the unconsciousness. Female patients may require catheter drainage, using a silastic balloon self-retaining catheter (Fig. 7.6), may be needed. Should this be necessary the precautions against urinary infection mentioned in Chapter 5 must be observed.

Whether the patient is male or female it is highly desirable that effective

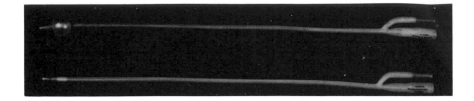

Fig. 7.6. A silastic balloon catheter.

nursing measures which avoid any internal device inside the urethra and urinary bladder be given a trial first; if catheterization can be avoided, urinary infection, with its serious sequelae, is less likely.

Nutrition

In normal health a sedentary male worker requires about 2,500 calories a day; this varies with the size of the body and endocrinal balance. Protein intake should be about 80 grammes.

The unconscious patient performs little or no physical activity apart from maintaining vital function such as respiration, peristalsis, and cardiac movements, but his calorie requirements are increased because of the healing process the body must carry out as a result of trauma, or surgical intervention, or disease. This means that the patient's calorie requirements are greater than those of a sedentary worker. A much larger quantity of protein must be supplied.

The unconscious patient will require about 2,800 calories. A protein, high calorie diet can be given intravenously, but when possible, an intragastric diet is given.

The dietary needs of the patient, who is unconscious, must be carefully assessed. The help of the therapeutic dietician or a specialist in parenteral and oral nutrition should be sought. It is possible to either under-feed or overfeed the patient, and to supply the wrong elements in the food. Frequent weight estimation, using special scales which weigh the bed and the occupant, is ideal. Blood chemistry must be analysed at regular intervals.

Diets in intragastric tube feeding

1 *Complan (Glaxo Ltd.)*. This is a patent food prepared especially for the purpose of feeding patients when normal diet is not possible. It is simple

to use and requires only to be dissolved in water; it contains all the constituents of a good diet (except roughage) in balanced proportions.

One pound of Complan equals:

Protein   140 grammes (574 calories)
Fat   74 grammes (681 calories)
Carbohydrate   200 grammes (820 calories)
Total   2,075 calories.

2   *Fluid diet*. Alternatively, a fluid diet can consist of combinations of dried milk, whole milk, Casilan, butter, eggs, sugar, salt, beef broth, vitamin syrup and iron compounds to make up a balanced diet with the items in balanced proportions. The therapeutic dietician is mainly concerned with providing a suitable diet, but the nurse must be fully aware of the needs of the patient.

3   *Liquidized normal diet*. This requires the use of an electrical food liquidizer. A whole normal diet, such as would be fed to a conscious person of similar age and weight as the patient using a knife, fork and spoon, is liquidized. The resultant fluid is then diluted with water to make sufficient feeds each of six fluid ounces (170 ml) in quantity.

The advantage of this system is that it overcomes the tendency to persistent diarrhoea and distension of abdomen that may be present in patients fed entirely on patent food. The patient who is conscious and on intragastric feeds gains psychological uplift when he knows that he is eating the same food as in normal circumstances.

Method of tube feeding

Feeding by tube is done at two or four-hourly intervals. The total dietary needs are divided into equal feeds to the required number. Extra quantities of water are given at feed times. During the first twenty-four hours the patient's fluid intake should be limited in order to avoid raising intracranial pressure. The prevention of dehydration is also important and this is more likely to happen in a patient who perspires a great deal; a balance must be achieved between intake and output. Thirst will cause the patient to be restless.

The intragastric tube can be passed with the patient in either the lateral or recumbent position; the nasal route is usually the most convenient. The nostrils are cleansed before passing the tube.

The main hazard to the patient is that the tube may be passed into the larynx and trachea instead of the oesophagus, and the position must be checked before passing any food down the tube. In most patients the entry of the tube into the larynx will cause coughing and cyanosis; it is then necessary to withdraw it and insert it correctly. When the tube has been passed correctly, further checks can be made by: (a) immersing the proximal end of the tube in water, when, if there are no bubbles, all is well; (b) aspirating some fluid from the tube with a syringe and testing the reaction of the fluid. If strongly acid, the tube is in the stomach. Finally, the graduated glass funnel is connected to the tube and the feed is given, at body temperature, a small quantity at a time. This is followed by some water. The intragastric tube may be left *in situ* for several feeds if it is flushed through with clean water each time. A once-daily change at least is essential.

If the patient's nutrition is adequate there need be no loss of weight or dehydration.

Maintenance of airway

Many surgeons carry out tracheostomy as a routine measure on patients who are likely to be unconscious for some days. Others prefer to avoid this procedure, as tracheostomy has its complications. There is no doubt that nursing and suction of the respiratory passages is simplified when tracheostomy has been performed. With tracheostomy, an endotracheal tube may be inserted.

Tracheostomy

A tracheostomy is a surgical opening into the trachea just below the larynx; a metal, polythene or rubber tube is inserted into the opening to keep it open.

Tracheostomy is performed on unconscious patients:
1   when the airway is obstructed by damage to the facial bones, tongue or larynx;
2   when the volume of respiration is inadequate to oxygenate the blood and prevent anoxia of the brain cells, and intermittent positive pressure ventilation (IPPV) is needed;
3   in elderly patients, particularly those with chronic bronchitis and bronchiectasis;
4   in chest infection when a possible complication arises if coughing is inadequate to clear the respiratory passages.
5   For the removal of secretions gathering in the trachea and bronchi and

obstructing the passage of air in the unconscious patient or when the cough reflex is absent.

When tracheostomy has not been performed, the nursing position must be in the semi-prone position, with the head lowered so that secretions gravitate out of the throat and mouth (Figs. 7.3 and 7.7).

It is frequently the only way of saving life; the procedure is also performed to improve ventilation of the lungs as part of treatment, although it is not essential for the survival of the patient.

SUCTION

Whether or not tracheostomy has been performed, frequent suction of the throat and trachea maintains the air passages clear of secretions, and eases the breathing in patients who, because the swallowing reflex is depressed, cannot carry out the normal swallowing action of the conscious individual clearing his throat.

An efficient suction machine is essential. It is connected to a soft rubber catheter with a bore large enough to clear blood clots and vomitus. It may be passed through the nasal cavity or mouth or tracheostomy tube. The catheter should be sterile if it is to enter the trachea.

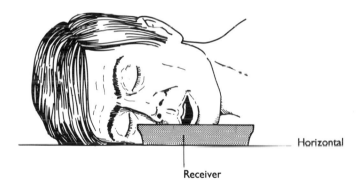

Horizontal

Receiver

Fig. 7.7. Drainage of the nose and throat of an unconscious patient.

Management of the tracheostomy tube

TYPES OF TUBE

Tubes may be either cuffed or uncuffed.

(a) Cuffed tube (Fig. 7.8). These are used to block off the upper respiratory passages so that the only entrance to the trachea is via the tube. After the tube has been inserted the cuff is inflated.

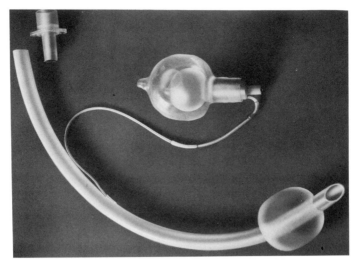

Fig. 7.8. A Lanz endotracheal tube with controlled pressure cuff. (Photograph supplied by Extracorporeal Medical Specialities, Inc., King of Prussia, Pa., U.S.A.

CARE OF THE TUBE

The tracheostomy tube and opening is the only portal of entry for air to reach the patient's lungs. Constant supervision is necessary to ensure that the tube does not become obstructed by sputum, and cause asphyxia. The tube is changed for a fresh one every second day; a replacement tube and tracheal dilator must always be ready for emergencies. The inside of the tube becomes crusted and requires thorough cleansing and sterllization.

Before removing a tube for replacement the pharynx must be cleared of secretions, via the mouth, with suction apparatus in order to prevent the secretions running down the trachea when the tube is taken out.

The wound (that is, the tracheostomy opening) 'must be dressed; nonadherent gauze against the tissues, surrounds the tube. The dressing technique is similar to that for any wound dressing. The main hazard to the patient, after asphyxia has been considered, is infection via the tube and wound.

Patient care

The patient with a tracheostomy tube in position has specific problems:
1   Communication. If the patient is conscious the presence of the tube and diversion of air away from the larynx means that the patient cannot talk, but if a finger is placed over the opening it may enable the patient to speak.

A writing pad and pencil, however, should be provided for more complex messages, but most needs should be anticipated by the nurse; experience and simple signals are often all that are needed.

2   Feeding. In the immediate post-operative phase the patient may find swallowing difficult, and intragastric tube feeding may be needed.

3   Mouth and nasal care. As the nasal cavities are not used for the passage of air they may become encrusted. They will require cleansing several times a day. The mouth requires full nursing care to prevent infection that would descend the tube.

4   Antibiotic cover. The surgeon may order antibiotics to prevent any infection that might retard the treatment of the patient.

5   Humidification of the inspired air. The patient's breathing through a tracheostomy tube does not use the normal physiological method of warming the air as it passes through the nasal cavities and pharynx. For optimal comfort and function, therefore, the air or oxygen that passes into the tracheostomy tube should be warmed and moistened. This may be done by using an atomizer or a humidifier. Both maintain a consistently humid environment for the patient. A patent tracheostomy mask that carries the humidifier air to the tracheostomy tube is also available.

6   Suction. To maintain the trachea and bronchi free of obstructive fluid secretions regular suction and clearing of the passages is essential. The removal of secretions is a skill that the nursing staff must acquire. An efficient suction machine is a necessary piece of apparatus near the patient's bedside. Sterile endotracheal catheters are used. These have openings in the side and end. Slight angulation on these catheters assists in directing them into the mouth and pharynx and for suction via the tube. They are used only once before resterilization or discarding.

The method of suction is as follows:

(a)   The catheter is connected via a tube and glass connection to the suction machine. The power of suction must be adequate to clear secretions only. Too powerful suction may collapse the lung.

(b)   The diameter of the catheter must be half that of the diameter of the tracheostomy tube opening. Too large a catheter would block the tracheostomy tube and cause asphyxia.

(c)   Hand washing by the nurse is essential before handling the sterile catheters.

(d)   The catheter is nipped by the fingers and held closed for the whole of the entry of the tube. It is released at the start of withdrawal, and secretions are sucked out on the return route.

(e)   The catheter is passed down the trachea beyond the bifurcation of the bronchi. When one bronchus has been cleared the catheter is passed into the other bronchus. Other helpers should tilt the patient towards the side to be cleared so that the catheter will enter the lowest brocnhus.

(f)   The catheter is handled with firm purposeful movements. 'Jiggling' it serves no purpose.

(g)   There is no set interval between suction treatments. The more copious the secretions the more frequent should be the suction of the patient, and vice versa. The noise of respiration will usually indicate the need for action. It is practicable to carry out suction at the same time as respiratory physiotherapy. Any secretions dislodged by physiotherapy can thus be aspirated.

Intermittent positive pressure ventilation

Using the IPPV system, air (plus oxygen, if necessary) is forced in and sucked out of the respiratory passages by means of either a cuffed tracheostomy tube or a cuffed endotracheal tube inserted via the mouth or nose, at a rate and in an amount to maintain normal pulmonary ventilation.

The advantages of this system are that the volume and rate of inspiration and expiration and the contents of the gases can be controlled accurately. Oxygen is given via the machine.

IPPV machines

The most important requirements of these machines are reliability and simplicity, as they are used by many people of limited mechanical ability. The more complex the machine, the more skilled must be the technician controlling it, and the main problem of any complex apparatus in hospital is that instruction in its use must be given to a large number of people, including all the grades of medical staff, nursing staff, and lay personnel. This often involves a massive training and teaching programme to ensure complete safety of the patient. The instruction manuals related to the machinery must form part of the equipment.

Many types of machine are available for intermittent positive pressure ventilation. All these machines vary in design, merits and disadvantages, and all are constantly being modified and improved. It is not possible, therefore, to give a definitive description of the method of using a particular machine. It is the duty of every member of the staff of a department where such a machine is likely to be used to become familiar with it before it is needed and a training schedule must exist. A regular maintenance routine by the hospital engineering staff is important. Both electrical and manual operation must be possible.

In using ventilation machines the first problem is to locate the controls and then to select a suitable rate of respiration. These are:

For an adult   12–16 per minute
For a child   20 per minute
For an infant   30 per minute

After this it is necessary to find the tidal volume appropriate for the rate; this is related to the weight of the patient. According to the respiratory efficiency of the patient and of the equipment, it will be necessary to modify, but these modifications are the responsibility of the doctor.

Once the rate and volume required are set, the machine can be connected to the patient's tracheostomy tube and intermittent positive pressure ventilation started. The patient must be constantly supervised; a warning light must also be set to shine and a bell to ring if the machine stops.

The complications and hazards of this form of care are:

1   A fall in blood pressure may occur soon after the process is started. In most patients this quickly readjusts.

2   Inadequate volume or rate. These may lead to anoxia and cyanosis. In some machines it may be difficult to set volume and rate accurately.

3   Dependence on the equipment. Weaning from the apparatus, when all is again normal, takes a long time. In some patients it can be switched off when no longer needed, but others require two or three days to adjust themselves, and still others need short periods, slightly increased each day over many days, before they can finally dispense with the assistance of the machine. Everything depends on the patient's condition, and we must constantly remind ourselves that every patient is an individual.

Drugs

The following drugs may be ordered by the doctor:

1   *Respiratory inhalants*

Breathing may be assisted by the use of inhalants which dissolve tenacious bronchial secretions and improve respiration.

2   *Antibiotics*

The doctor may wish to provide the patient with a broad-spectrum antibiotic cover to prevent respiratory or urinary infection retarding progress.

3   *Mineral elements and vitamins*

These are used to supplement the diet. When prolonged vomiting or diarrhoea has occurred the doctor may order sodium or potassium to counteract electrolyte imbalance; these items may be given by the parenteral route depending upon the reports of the daily blood-chemistry analysis.

4   *Urinary antiseptics*

These may be ordered when frequent catheterization is necessary, in order to combat urinary infection.

Physiotherapy

The physiotherapist has a part to play in helping in the survival of the unconscious patient. She can help by percussing the thorax of the patient when he is turned, the aim being to clear plugs of mucus that may obstruct the bronchioles. Chest percussion is often complemented with tracheal suction. The physiotherapist also helps applying passive movements to all the joints of the body in order to try to prevent stiffness and deformity.

Return to consciousness

The term 'unconsciousness' suggests that the patient is apathetic and immobile; this is frequently not so. Many patients can be unconscious but also restless, noisy, obstreperous and difficult to manage. Their care requires patience and ingenuity. A full bladder or rectum, or severe thirst can all cause distress, which results in restlessness or noisiness.

Restless movement or shouting are not to the detriment of the patient, provided he is protected from injury, and they may even improve his condition. The nursing and physiotherapy staff work to prevent stasis of tissues and lungs; the noisy, restless patient contributes to this effort and reduces the need.

The patient can be restrained from falling out of bed by the use of nets, even if such ideas are repugnant to the nursing staff. The most logical place for the patient's mattress is on the floor; he can then fall no further. Cot sides without a net are frequently useless, as the patient can fling himself over them, or he can bruise or tear his skin unless the cot sides are padded. The noise from the patient is distressing to others, and a side ward is the most suitable place for his care, provided he is under constant supervision.

The patient who returns to partial consciousness in hospital can be frightened, confused and worried, by his strange surroundings. As consciousness returns, the sitting position will reduce confusion. Sedation is usually discouraged, unless the patient is completely unmanageable, as it is important to know the level of his consciousness.

Rehabilitation

The recovery of consciousness, does not mean the end of the patient's problems. The effects of brain damage are related to the part of the brain which has been damaged and the seriousness of the lesion. If the damage is localized to a lobe of the cerebrum, unconsciousness is not inevitable, but there will be ensuing problems.

If the frontal lobes are the site of a lesion, there will be changes in the personality of the patient; damage to the temporal lobes will result in problems in storing new events to memory; an injury to one of the occipital lobes can cause loss of sight in an eye; cerebellar injuries will result in loss of coordination of limbs and problems of balance; paralysis is caused if the parietal lobes undergo damage. It is the two latter results which come within the frame of reference of this book.

It follows that the injury to the brain will take many forms and the results will be infinitely variable. Recovery may take many months and then may be incomplete.

The patient will, therefore, be a patient and under some form of medical or hospital care for a long time. His management follows the same pattern as that of patients discussed elsewhere in this book. For the management of the hemiplegic patient see Chapter 8. The patient with cerebellar damage will have similar problems to those with cerebral palsy which is discussed in Chapter 9.

Head injuries club

Hospitals which have neurological and trauma units for the management of patients with head injuries usually provide special facilities for the patient who is recovering from the long-term problems. This may take the form of premises with staff who provide day case care or residential facilities for the patient. Retraining is given in daily-living activities. Industrial, clerical or craft work, penmanship, speech therapy and social relationships are all facets of the work of the 'club'. All activities are related to the speed and ability of the patient as he recovers.

8 : Adult Hemiplegia and the Geriatric Patient

Relevant anatomy and physiology

The normal functioning of any part of the body requires that the blood is passed to the heart and lungs for re-oxygenation. Normally the blood is confined within the tubes called the blood vessels; arteries, arterioles, capillaries and veins. Transference of 'life essentials' from the flowing blood to the tissue cells and return of waste products from the tissue cells to the bloodstream occurs through the walls of capillaries (Fig. 8.1).

Capillaries are elastic, malleable, resilient tubes capable of expanding and contracting according to the amount of blood being pumped into them at any given moment. They determine the variability of blood pressure which rises sufficiently but no higher than is essential in response to transient extra activity within the tissue and which quickly falls to 'normal' when the extra pressure demand has passed.

In youth and health this system functions well. Thus we can lift heavy weights, run or swim great distances at speed, consume ponderous meals and demonstrate extreme anger without harming ourselves. In good health some of these activities may even improve the state of the tissues: the sedentary person is often less fit than the vigorous.

As we increase in age and maltreat our bodies both by inadequate exercise and with excessive food, alcohol, nicotine or other toxic substance, the quality of our blood vessels deteriorates and instead of the tubes being elastic and resilient they become increasingly stiff and eventually brittle. Linked with this hardening of the blood vessels, there is an increase in the pressure of blood within them which is then maintained at a higher level than is necessary even when the body is at rest. It follows that when stresses, emotional or physical, are applied to the body the tubes are unable to receive the increased volume and pressure without breaking as a result of their brittleness.

As the bursting of the blood vessel is most likely to occur within the cranial cavity the result is usually catastrophic to the central nervous system. Such a disaster creates a 'space-occupying lesion' either intra- or extra-dural haematoma as described on page 173 and this results in an upper motor neurone lesion as described on page 152.

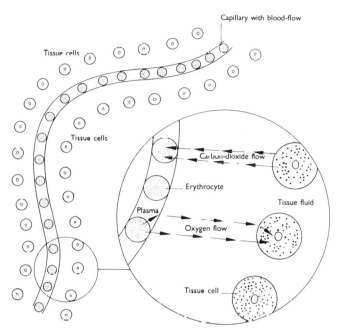

Fig. 8.1. Internal respiration and the transfer of products from the blood to tissues.

ADULT HEMIPLEGIA

Aetiology

Hemiplegia in the adult may occur for a variety of causes, but the over whelming majority are due to cerebrovascular accidents (strokes). Other causes include injury, syphilis, abscesses, tumours, emboli, thrombosis and aneurysms. In addition to the hemiplegia, the patient may have aphasia, if the dominant hemisphere is affected, and varying degrees of mental and emotional impairment.

Treatment

In the early stages, it is important to avoid contractures in the paralysed limb and these must be positioned correctly; every joint must be put through a full range of movement at least once daily (preferably more often) there is considerable evidence that adequate early physiotherapy and positioning the joints can favourably influence the ultimate pattern of reflex activity and the ultimate function of the limb.

If left untreated, a leg paralysed from an upper motor neurone lesion, tends to assume a characteristic position—flexed and adducted at the hip, flexed at the knee and the foot in equino varus. (Fig. 8.2). In the arm, the classical position is adduction and internal rotation at the shoulder, flexion at the elbow, wrist and fingers and pronation of the forearm. Usually the arm is more affected than the leg and arm recovery is less complete.

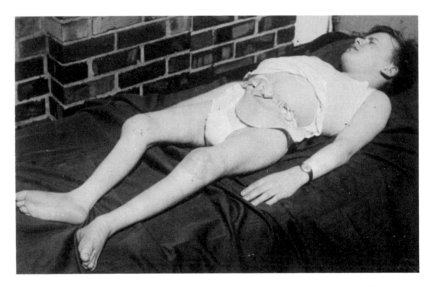

Fig. 8.2. A paralysed leg to show the posture of the hip, knee and foot.

'Strokes' may be of all degrees from a transient impairment of speech, to complete hemiplegia with loss of consciousness and death within a few hours.

Prognosis obviously depends on the pathological basis—a massive cerebral haemorrhage in a hypertensive patient is likely to be rapidly fatal. A transient vasospasm in a normotensive patient carries an excellent prognosis.

Medical treatment will include the control of blood pressure, and if the patient is unconscious, the usual nursing routines (q.v.).

As already indicated, positioning of the paralysed limbs and if necessary, the appropriate splinting for a drop wrist or drop foot, will be needed. Later on, physiotherapy will be needed. Occasionally specific orthopaedic appliances such as a walking caliper to control a collapsing knee (Fig. 8.3) or a toe-spring for a drop foot, (Fig. 8.4) may be needed to enable a patient to walk. Operative intervention is only occasionally required but the following procedures may be needed:

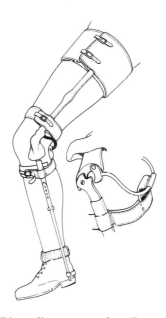

Fig. 8.3.   A walking caliper to control a collapsing knee and a knee cage.

For the arm:
1   Elongation of finger flexor tendons where the fingers are tightly clenched into the palm (Fig. 8.5).
2   Transplant of flexor tendons for 'wrist drop' (Fig. 8.6).
3   Release of pronator muscles.
4   Elongation of biceps.
5   Elongation of shoulder adductors and medial rotators.
    For the leg:
1   Transplant of half the tibialis anterior to the outer side of the foot for an inverted foot (stirrup procedure) (Fig. 8.7 a and b).
2   Transplant of the tibialis posterior muscle to the anterior aspect of the

Fig. 8.4.   A toe-spring for a drop-foot.

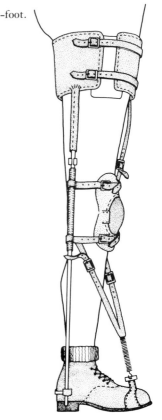

Fig. 8.5.(a)   Elongation of flexor tendons
in a spastic hand.

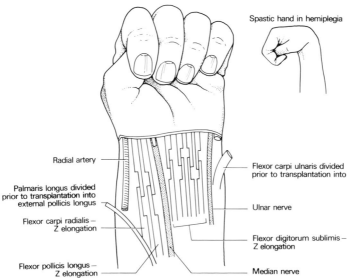

Spastic hand in hemiplegia

Radial artery

Palmaris longus divided
prior to transplantation into
external pollicis longus

Flexor carpi radialis —
Z elongation

Flexor pollicis longus —
Z elongation

Flexor carpi ulnaris divided
prior to transplantation into

Ulnar nerve

Flexor digitorum sublimis —
Z elongation

Median nerve

(b)

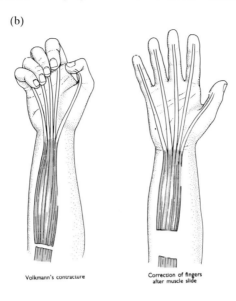

Volkmann's contracture   Correction of fingers after muscle slide

Fig. 8.5.(b) Correction of Volkmann's contracture.

(a)   (b)

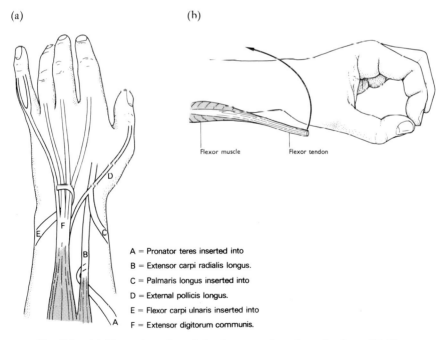

Flexor muscle   Flexor tendon

A = Pronator teres inserted into
B = Extensor carpi radialis longus.
C = Palmaris longus inserted into
D = External pollicis longus.
E = Flexor carpi ulnaris inserted into
F = Extensor digitorum communis.

Fig. 8.6. (a) Transplantation of the finger tendons for wrist drop. (b) Transplantation of the flexor tendon.

(a)   (b)   (c)

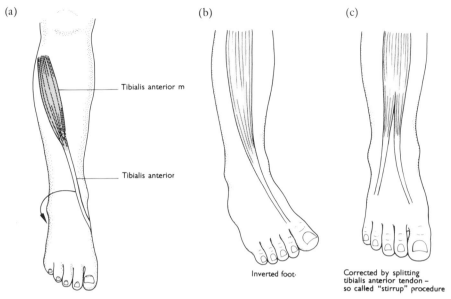

Tibialis anterior m

Tibialis anterior

Inverted foot·

Corrected by splitting
tibialis anterior tendon –
so called "stirrup" procedure

Fig. 8.7. (a) Splitting the tibialis anterior for correcting varus deformity. Half of the tendon is transplanted to the outer side of the foot. (b) Stirrup procedure for correction of inverted foot.

foot and elongation of the calcaneal tendon for equino-varus deformity of the foot (Fig. 8.8 a–d).

3 Eggers' operation for flexion deformity of the knee (Fig. 8.9 a and b).

4 Mizouno's operation for flexion and adduction deformity of the hip (Fig. 8.10).

The success of all these procedures depends on correct after-treatment, re-educating the transferred muscles to undertake a new function. They are unlikely to be successful if the patient cannot cooperate.

The management of the hemiplegic patient

As the hemiplegia may be either in an uncomplicated form or complicated by:

1 two lesions affecting both sides of the brain; 2 hemianaesthesia; 3 hemianopia; 4 aphasia; 5 apraxia; 6 agnosia; 7 emotional disturbance and alteration of personality; 8 intellectual impairment.

Careful assessment of the total problems of the patient is essential. A full neurological and clinical examination must be performed to estimate the following:

1   The total motor function of the affected limbs with grading of the degree of muscle function in detail. 2   Reflex action at abdomen, elbow, knee, ankle and foot. 3   Perception—ability to recognize objects by sight, touch, taste or smell. 4   Cognition—awareness of events and activities. 5   Comprehension—understanding what is said and what is meant. 6   Communication—the ability to convey needs and ideas. 7   Memory— to recall dates and personal events. 8   Orientation—an awareness of surroundings.

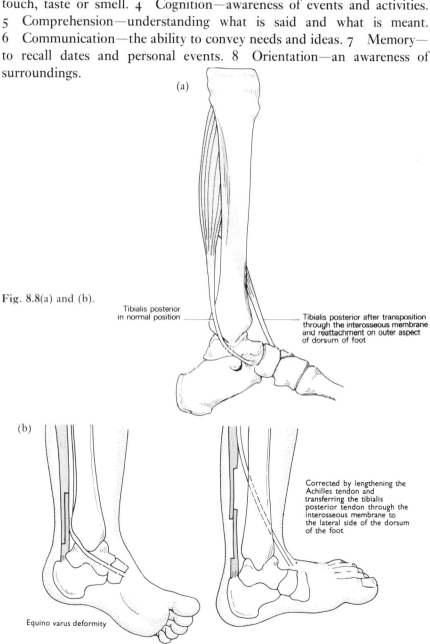

(a)

Fig. 8.8(a) and (b).

Tibialis posterior in normal position

Tibialis posterior after transposition through the interosseous membrane and reattachment on outer aspect of dorsum of foot

(b)

Corrected by lengthening the Achilles tendon and transferring the tibialis posterior tendon through the interosseous membrane to the lateral side of the dorsum of the foot

Equino varus deformity

(c)   (d)   (f)

(e)

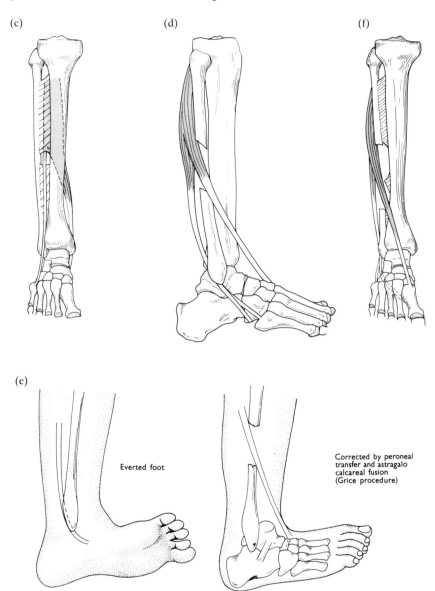

Everted foot

Corrected by peroneal
transfer and astragalo
calcareal fusion
(Grice procedure)

Fig.8.8.   (a) and (b) Medial views of the tibialis posterior transplant for equino-
varus deformity. (c) Tibialis posterior transfer for equino-varus deformity;
anterior view. (d) Transplant of peroneal tendons for valgus foot lateral view
combined with subastragaloid fusion using the resected fibula as grafts. (e) Grice
procedure for correction of everted foot. (f) Peroneous transfer for valgus foot
usually combined with subastragaloid fusion using the resected portion of the
fibual anterior view.

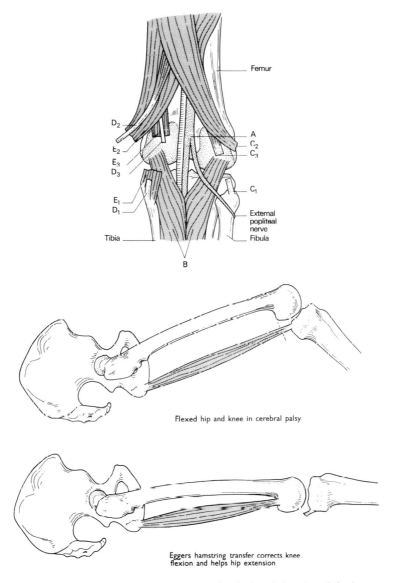

Fig. 8.9. (a) and (b) Egger's operation for flexion deformity of the knee.

It is necessary to find out which areas of the brain are affected. Such knowledge is relevant to the treatment and prognosis of the condition. A total evaluation of functional loss is carried out. The ability to stand, walk, talk, dress, use the toilet and the amount of recovery which will be necessary to achieve these abilities is estimated.

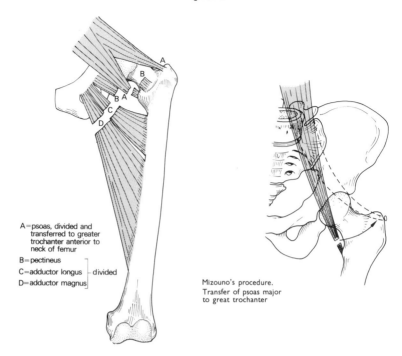

A=psoas, divided and
transferred to greater
trochanter anterior to
neck of femur

B=pectineus

C=adductor longus ⎱ divided

D=adductor magnus ⎰

Mizouno's procedure.
Transfer of psoas major
to great trochanter

Fig. 8.10. (a) and (b) Mizouno's operation for spastic dislocation of the hip. This is easily done through a medial approach with the hip flexed, abducted and externally rotated.

The patient's environment

In hemiplegic management, as in other conditions, the social background influences the patient's recovery. If the home circumstances are suitable, the discharge from hospital can be sooner and this is usually best for the patient. When the patient is to return to an uninhabited home his stay in hospital must be prolonged and there is a danger that the patient may become institutionalized; that is, totally dependent upon the hospital and staff with fear of departure from the institution to home.

Hemiplegic management particularly requires full coordination between the hospital and the community.

Psychological distress

The stroke which caused the hemiplegia may be seen and felt as 'the last straw' to an ageing patient. Recent personal history may have included

1 retirement from active professional life and a feeling of being unwanted,
2 the need to adjust to being at home, losing the companionship of colleagues.
3 boredom and inability to fill time,
4 bereavement, due to loss of the wife or husband,
5 dependence upon children with an impression of being in the way.

Thus the patient who may have already been partly demoralized by some of the above is often in a depressed state when he enters hospital. The staff responsible for his care must be aware of this and should study and correct the patient's mental attitudes. He may feel that he is approaching the death he has seen occur to many of his contemporaries in recent years. This mental depression is a major problem of managing any hemiplegic patient. It is necessary to convince him that improvement and recovery can and does occur in many paralysed patients. Even if he does not gain full use of his limbs and a return of speech, it is still possible to return to an interesting and happy life in the community and out of hospital. The patient's relatives and friends must be as optimistic as the staff of the hospital. A very important aspect of this is the need to see positive steps towards his recovery being taken. Apathy must not arise.

INCONTINENCE AND DISTRESS

The elderly patient who has been fastidious in dress, grooming, personal hygiene and modesty finds the problem of soiled clothing and bed-sheets embarrassing and distressing. The misery of this problem may exceed all others.

Conscientious nursing is necessary to relieve the distress. Positive planning to move the patient on to the toilet, using a special chair, in time to control the timing of evacuation of the bowel or bladder; condom and polythene receptacles (see page 138) and the judicious use of suppositories (see page 137) on the patient will avoid the soiling of clothing or bed.

Again the mental attitude of the patient must be understood. A discussion of the problem with the patient to explain that incontinence happens with his ailment and that control of bladder and rectum will return.

Sloppy dress, such as slippers and dressing gown, must be discouraged as soon as feasible. Both male and female patients should be encouraged to reach their normal level of grooming and cosmetic management.

The problems of the hemiplegic patient

It is difficult to analyse the finer problems of the patient without the actual experience of being paralysed down one side of the body. This section is a breakdown of the hemiplegic state.

There is a loss of initiative and memory accompanied by confusion and a tendency to emotional distress which cannot be controlled. Because of loss of feeling on the affected side the patient is unable to interpret directional instructions; thus forwards, backwards, sideways to right or left are terms which are easily misunderstood.

As the nerve tracts which keep the brain informed of the position of joints, muscles and ultimately the limb do not function, the patient is unable to estimate the posture of his affected limbs without visual examination and feeling with his unaffected limb. Thus the patient may appear to spend a great deal of time studying and prodding the affected limbs. As there is loss of control of the lateral half of the trunk as well as the affected limbs, balancing upright in a chair, moving the buttocks or turning over in bed cannot be achieved without training. Lying horizontal in a moving vehicle, such as on a stretcher or in an ambulance can create a terror of falling because of the inability to use the limbs for balance and protection.

Putting on garments is difficult and frustrating. Movements to thread sleeves on to arms or trousers on to legs are hard to achieve without help and training. Fine movements in fastening zips, buttons, or clips with one hand take a lot of time particularly if the unaffected arm is the left one in a right-handed patient.

Communication by speech or writing is a severe problem. Converting thoughts into speech or print may not be possible. Loss of use of hands used in speech gestures is frustrating. Inability to communicate particularly in an intelligent patient, may result in temperamental outbursts.

Teamwork

As with all patient management, the aged patient requires the combined efforts of many hospital workers. The geriatric physician is a doctor who has made a particular study of the ageing patient and he coordinates the activities of nursing staff, physiotherapists, occupational therapists, medical social workers, speech therapists, therapeutic dietician, pharmacitst, district nurses and the patient's own general practitioner. The care of this patient requires dedication by all members of the team.

Urinary infections in the elderly

Surveys of elderly people show that many suffer from urinary tract infections. Females are more likely to be affected than males and it is considered that the shorter urethra of the female terminating in the folded moist vulva may cause this.

Many sufferers from urinary infection in non-hospitalized elderly people do not attend for medical treatment.

Stagnation in the urinary flow can contribute to the problem. This may be caused by a sluggish peristaltic wave caused by senile deterioration of the body. Enlargement of the prostate gland, and any other condition such as a diverticulum or cystocoele in the wall of the bladder (Fig. 8.11) which may cause conditions which are favourable to multiplication, after successful invasion of micro-organisms. Another contributory factor may be the lowered resistance to infection which may be present in anaemic people.

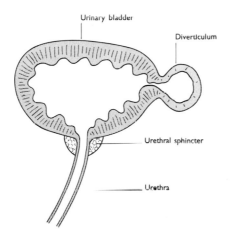

Fig. 8.11. A diverticulum of the urinary bladder.

DIAGNOSIS OF URINARY INFECTION

An essential part of the treatment of urinary infection is identification of the organism which is causing the problem. As urinary infection is often related to incontinence, it follows that a fresh midstream specimen must be collected for pathological examination. Commonly, *Escherichia coli* is found. The presence of micro-organisms in the urinary system, and this cystitis or pyelonephritis will aggravate the difficulty of which the cerebro-vascular accident patient has in controlling his bladder and thus incontinence of urine often ensues. When the infecting micro-organism is recognized and the specific antibiotic given the urinary infection will clear provided there are no gross anatomical abnormalities of the urinary system. If control of the infection occurs at the same time as improvement of the cerebrovascular state, the incontinence can be resolved.

PYELONEPHRITIS

An infection of the kidney which may be haematogenous (blood-borne); ascending from the bladder to kidneys via the ureters; or from the bladder via the lymphatic chain. There is acute inflammation of the kidneys.

Symptoms and signs of pyelonephritis

There is severe pain in the loins, local tenderness over the kidneys, pyrexia, malaise, headache, rigors, frequency and painful micturition.

Examination of the urine reveals a sediment of debris when it is allowed to stand in a specimen glass. Albumen and blood will be present on testing and pus cells will be seen on microscopic examination.

The patient will be apathetic about his environment, constantly drowsy and ultimately 'uraemic'. If the condition progresses there may be ventricular failure of the heart, dyspnoea, pulmonary oedema, and death.

Treatment of urinary infection

Correct antibiotic therapy is related to the number of micro-organisms seen in the laboratory specimen and to the sensitivity of the organisms to specific antibiotics. There is not a 'universal' antibiotic or drug for cystitis and it is wise to use the precise antibiotic which is specific for the particular organisms. By testing the sensitivity of the organism to a wide variety of drugs the correct antibiotic can be selected. A combination of antibiotics may be required and the doctor will usually seek the advice of the pathologist about this.

It is essential to appreciate that antibiotics and urinary antiseptics, if used for an unnecessarily long period, can result in permanent kidney damage and also infection of the gastro-intestinal tract by resistant organisms.

It is also important to realize that antibiotics may cause side effects. These side effects on elderly patients with cerebrovascular problems are likely to be serious. Skin rashes, gastric distress, peripheral nerve lesions are possible and the nurse must observe the patient on antibiotics and chemotherapy for such complications. Any complaint of skin irritation, indigestion and flatulence, tingling or numbness, ringing in the ear, deafness or other new and unusual symptoms must be reported to the doctor in charge of the patient.

To avoid these side effects it is the practice to alternate courses of chemotherapy with courses of urinary antiseptics. Thus ten days on one followed by ten days on the other will reduce the possibility of side effects. In this way pyelonephritis, which may be chronic and persistent, can be controlled and relapse prevented. Another advantage of this method is that smaller doses of the drugs will be effective. Pathological examination of urinary specimens, collected frequently, will prove or disprove this.

FLUID INTAKE AND OUTPUT

All elderly patients require careful recording of the amounts of fluid they ingest and excrete when infection is present. When infection is present the attendant pyrexia, confusion, toxicity and dehydration require careful regulation of the fluid intake and resultant output. The daily intake when a balance is estimated should exceed the output by about 500 ml and two litres per day of urinary excretion is the aim of management.

This is difficult to achieve in an elderly patient who will not drink. Good nursing management requires constant unremitting persuasion so that all the nursing attendants manage to make the patient drink some fluid at every nursing attention.

When it is not possible to reach the 2.5 litre intake by the oral route the parenteral pathway using intravenous infustin must be the alternative.

THE MANAGEMENT OF INCONTINENCE

The volume of fluid required as part of the antibiotic, chemotherapy and urinary antiseptics will increase or create the problems of incontinence. The use of the condom device (see Chapter 5 page 138 for the male and an indwelling balloon catheter (see Chapter 5, page 141) for the female is required.

It may be necessary to perform catheterization as a diagnostic measure on either male or female patient (a) when a sterile specimen of urine must be obtained for culture of micro-organisms in selecting the relevant anti-biotics (b) when the patient is in coma and cannot cooperate in supplying a midstream specimen (c) in acute urinary retention (d) to estimate residual urine after voluntary voiding. Catheterization must only be performed under the highest standard of a septic technique possible and interference must always be avoided, if this is feasible.

A major problem in the management of the confused geriatric patient is that of interference with the urinary device by the patient. Communication is often difficult and persuading the patient not to pull out the balloon catheter or remove the condom device requires much nursing tolerance. It is difficult for any elderly person to accept interference with their 'private parts' without objection.

Drug medication in the elderly

Developments in pharmacology in recent years have produced a range of drugs of far greater effectiveness than has previously existed. These drugs are effective and potent. They include: antibiotics, chemothera-peutics, tranquillizers, antidepressives, diuretics, steroids and synthetic drugs, which have an atropine-like effect. It is often the very efficiency of these drugs which is a danger to the elderly patient. When such a wide range of drugs is available it is essential that time is taken to assess the specific drugs which will benefit a particular patient. There is always a danger of human error both by the doctor who prescribes, and the nurse who administers drugs to older patients. There is also the probability that any staff who are involved in managing elderly patients are busy, probably overworked people without the time available to spend in considering the precise needs of the patient. Thus drugs may be prescribed because time is not available to allay the anxiety of a patient by communication in simple terms spoken slowly and clearly. Drugs may be given for far longer than is necessary. It is the function of nursing staff, particularly when dealing with aged patients, to be aware of the optimum period of administration of a drug and to keep the doctor-in-charge fully informed of the range of drugs, the dosage, the length of time the patient has been receiving the drug. The elderly are particularly vulnerable to adverse reactions to drugs. Often the kidneys of old patients do not function effectively and drugs will accummulate in the tissues more quickly because of impaired circulation in the brain due to poor cardiac function and decreased vascularity.

Examples of drugs used in the management of elderly patients

ANTIBIOTICS

These are a major factor in prolonging the life of many members of the population of all ages.

Their use and the ensuing rapid cure of many infections is a particular boon to the aged. Respiratory, cardiac, alimentary and urinary infections are all problems which may reduce the span of life in the geriatric patient. Without the antibiotics the mortality rate would be raised. Complications with antibiotics therapy occur in the elderly just as in any age group. Enquiry must always be made about allergy such as rashes, asthma, bronchospasm and previous antibiotic therapy. An allergic response to an antibiotic in an elderly patient can be fatal.

ANTIDEPRESSANT DRUGS

Amphetamine, phenelzine and transcyclopromine are drugs in this group and they are monoamine oxidase inhibitors. This means that these drugs in combination with some others such as imipramine may cause a severe hypertensive crisis. A similar reaction may be caused by eating cheese, yeast extract or beans in combination with the drugs which are monoamine oxidase inhibitors. Complaints of dizziness and palpitations must not be ignored in patients receiving these drugs.

ASPIRIN

Aspirin is effective and is still the most popular analgesic both to doctors and to patients who can buy it easily in the chemist's shop. It has certain disadvantages, however. It is composed of acetylsalicylic acid which is rapidly converted in the stomach to a corrosive which is salicylic acid. There is a high incidence of erosion of the stomach lining which can happen rapidly and result in serious bleeding. This is a tendency which can increase if the intake of vitamin 'C' into the patient is inadequate.

The elderly person who is on a poor diet, at home, because of apathy and loneliness, is most likely to be deficient in vitamin C. He is also the sufferer from chronic pains in joints, and chronic headaches, who is likely to consistently consume a high intake of aspirin.

Chronic bleeding, secondary to aspirin intake, is common in elderly people.

ATROPINE-LIKE DRUGS

Parkinsonism is a common condition among aged patients; it responds modestly well to drugs belonging to the belladonna drugs, tincture of belladonna, tincture of strammonium and synthetic atropine-like drugs such as benzhexol. These drugs tend to stimulate and there is a possibility of severe delirium and hallucinations in aged patients. It is necessary to start with very small doses which increase gradually.

BARBITURATES

Elderly patients are affected in unpredictable ways by the barbiturates As the kidneys do not function as efficiently as in younger patients there is a tendency for cumulative action to occur with resultant confusion, dorwsiness and distorted vision. The night problems for the nurse caring for such patients include the danger of the patient falling out of bed or disturbing others by wandering about.

DIGITALIS

Cardiac disease is often a part of ageing. Digoxin and digitalis are necessary in the management of elderly patients. Strict supervision of patients on these drugs is necessary to ensure that the drug is not over-effective and too large a dose being given. When overdosage has occurred, lowered appetite, headache, vomiting, bradycardia, dicrotic pulse and yellow vision may be present.

Cessation of the use of digitalis and treatment with vitamins and a diet rich in protein will cause a rapid improvement.

DIURETICS

Oral diuretics such as chlorothiazide, frusemide, bendrofluazide act upon the kidney tubules resulting in increased excretion of sodium and an increased output of urine.

Excretion of sodium also involves excretion of potassium and may result in a fall in potassium in the blood with a tendency to an increased ventricular rate and muscular weakness.

Doctors normally prescribe potassium chloride or other potassium salt to avoid this complication.

EPHEDRINE *and other sympathomimetic drugs*

These valuable bronchodilators also have a stimulant effect upon sphincter muscles. They are useful in the management of female patients with chronic bronchitis and stress incontinence. They are not suitable, in many case, for males with hypertension and retention of urine due to an enlarged prostrate gland.

TRANQUILLIZERS

These are of immense value in the management of psychotic and neurotic disorders. They have side effects such as hypothermia and hypotension which may be dangerous and lead to prolonged coma and death in elderly patients who are living in unheated or badly heated accommodation.

Speech problems

Dysphasia is one of the most serious complications of a stroke and many patients who have cerebrovascular accidents suffer from this.

There is, in all people, an interrelationship between mental imagery and words. Thus nouns such as 'table', 'chair' or 'spoon' conjure up transient pictures, in the mind, of the object named. This imagery applies also to complex and abstract words although without the precise mental picture-making; symbols are formed instead.

This same process applies in converting the written word into mental meaning. Thus the reception of the image-making process is via the eye and not the ear as in speech interpretation.

There are three parts to either form of communication:

1 Reception and transmission of the words, seen or heard, to the brain.

2 Conversion of the words into mental pictures.

3 Response either by spoken reply or facial expression. These are normally subjected to automatic internal monitoring.

Speech disorders in stroke patients may be the result of interruption of any of these processes.

As the speech area of the brain is in the dominant hemisphere, and this is the left in a right-handed person and right in a left-handed person a stroke affecting one side of the brain will create speech disorders in some patients and lesion of the opposite side will affect speech in others.

The functions of the speech therapist

1   *Establishing a means of communication.* The speech therapist can do much to improve the patient's ability to communicate with others (including nurses, doctors, physiotherapists and occupational therapists) and as a result, help to a marked extent with his treatment and management. Others may attempt to communicate but cannot achieve the level of communication of the speech therapist. Help is required from her in the early management of the patient.

2   *Assessing the problem.* It is necessary to know the extent and variety of dysphasia (see page 206). She will have a variety of aids to assist her in this including objects and pictures familiar to the patient.

3   *Re-education in understanding speech and phonation.* This will take the form of individual treatment and group therapy. All forms of communication are encouraged including speaking, singing, miming, writing and drawing.

Much of this is similar to the form of instruction given to children in school.

4   *Instruction of staff and relatives.* It is a common reaction of people who wish to talk to a patient who cannot speak to shout or use baby talk. There is no place for either method but communication with all patients is possible once the relevant method is found. Slow careful pronunciation as used in speaking to a foreigner is often successful.

All workers in the rehabilitation team must appreciate the frustrations of a patient who cannot speak. The patient can often full understand all which is said to him and around him yet is unable to respond. This can lead to anger and an unwanted rise in blood pressure.

As the initial symptoms of aphasia disappear, speech will improve and a more stable pattern of impairment which is acceptable to the patient and his relatives will evolve.

9 : Cerebral Palsy

Relevant applied anatomy and physiology

Nerve tissue is a soft delicate material which needs to be well protected by bony cavities, sheaths, membranes and fluids. Because it is so well protected the central nervous system is usually unaffected by the normal stresses and strains of living.

Before the protective coverings are properly formed however, in the prenatal, natal and neonatal phases, whilst the infant's skull and spine are still forming and growing, the central nervous system is vulnerable. The central nervous system may sustain injuries and scarring as the result of such catastrophes as infection, ischaemia, anoxia, biochemical disorders of its blood supply and simple traumatic bruising or crushing. Such injury is disastrous, particularly in the phase when the nervous tissue is forming and growing, because nerve cells do not regenerate, repair and replace themselves as efficiently as other tissues do. The end result of any form of the lesions mentioned is the formation of fibrous scar tissue in place of nervous tissue. Such tissue will not function, or contribute to the functions, which are normally carried out by nervous tissue namely initiation and transmission of impulses which travel over the brain, spinal cord and peripheral nerves via tracts or pathways. The inactive scar tissue replaces the living active nervous tissue and serves only to impede its function and interrupt its pathways. Indeed it may act as an irritant causing either further progressive loss of function or it may initiate abnormal impulses as in some forms of epilepsy. Thus infection, chemical interference from drugs, biochemical changes from metabolism or blood dyscrasia, ischaemia as a result of impairment of the blood flow, anoxia as the result of reduced oxygen supply, and injuries which affect the brain and spinal cord of the unborn or newly born infant can leave permanent, irreparable damage. There are many examples of such damage. The results will be related to the site of the damage. Thus any form of lesion may cause impaired vision, impaired hearing, motor or sensory loss of nerve supply to any part of the brain, spinal cord or body.

Recent progress in the knowledge of embryology, obstetrics and paediatrics indicates that many of the causes of such damage are likely to be preventable in the future and thus it is hoped that the number of patients who are so disabled will be greatly reduced.

Cerebral palsy in infancy

A large number of syndromes and included under this composite term, they are characterized by the fact that there is damage to the brain or parts of the brain, possibly associated with damage to the cervical spine as well. Both the causes of the damage and their anatomical localization are extremely variable, so it is not surprising that the number and variety of clinical syndromes is also very great. These conditions have one factor in common, that is that the child has impairment of muscle control of varying degree which is ultimately associated with spasticity of the muscles and hypertonicity (Fig. 9.1). However, even this fundamental definition is not adequate in very early infancy as the child may at first, have a flaccid paralysis and it is only as other parts of the nervous system mature that the paralysis assumes the classical spastic form.

Causes

There are many causes of cerebral palsy. It may be due to prenatal intrauterine effects, which in their turn may be of genetic origin. It may be due to toxic influences, to temporary placental ischaemia interfering with the nutrition of the developing central nervous system, or possibly may be due to various infections of the mother during pregnancy which may have passed the placental barrier and affect the child. Classically, syphilis was an example of a maternal infection which could affect the developing child, but we now know that a large number of other infections, virus diseases, toxic plasmosis, etc., may equally affect the child *in utero*.

Another group of causes is damage to the brain during the actual delivery. This may be because there is ischaemia or because there is actually a cerebral haemorrhage or excessive pressure on the head due to moulding, or pressure from the obstetrician's forceps, or from too rapid delivery in the case of breach presentation. In the immediate postnatal period there is some evidence that severe illness, failure to thrive, low blood pressure and malnutrition, may all lead to permanent interference with brain development. At a slightly older age infections, particularly of the central nervous system may of course, lead to cerebral defects. Equally, thrombophlebitis often associated with a severe marasmic illness, may lead to damage to the brain. Cerebral tumours, though relatively rare, and injury to the head in the postnatal period may also lead to the phenomenon of cerebral palsy and perhaps some cerebral palsy cases are due to non-accidental injuries of babies.

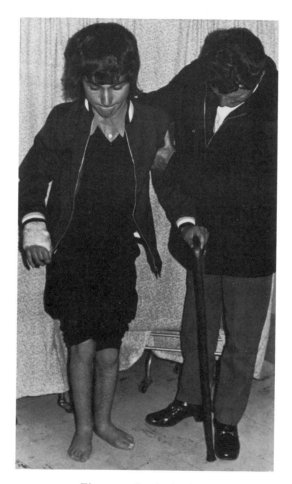

Fig. 9.1. Cerebral palsy.

Symptoms and signs

The clinical phenomena are of course, multitudinous. In the first place, the child may have a varying degree of mental impairment; however, in certain forms of cerebral palsy, particularly athetosis, it is usual for the child to be very intelligent. Certainly the average of their intelligence quotient is well up to normal but in other forms of cerebral palsy the intelligence is often below par and may on occasions, be very low indeed. Associated with evidence of damage to the brain there may be a varying degree of defect in the senses of vision and hearing. These may combine to give the impression that the child is more backward than he really is, and a certain number of quite intelligent children have been labelled as mentally deficient either because they were deaf or partly blind, and these may lead to great difficulties in the learning process. Therefore, in every instance the child's vision and hearing acuity should be carefully assessed by experts and corrected as far as possible. The cardinal feature of the disorder is a weakness or imperfect control of muscles associated ultimately with excessive tone and exaggerated reflex responses. There may be associated impairment of sensation and in particular, many of these children suffer from impairment of body image affecting the affected arm or leg. This is of great importance because our ability to put the limbs to any skilled use depends on us having an adequate awareness of their position and shape, their range of movement, their general configuration and so on. Measures directed purely to restoring muscle control, unless these are associated with adequate awareness of the limb as a whole, are not likely to lead to improvement in function. In addition to disorders of the skeletal muscle these children will often have problems in swallowing, chewing and breathing. As already stated, shortly after birth, the child will often be a 'floppy baby' and the tone in the limbs will be diminished. It will be noticed that the baby is less active than a normal baby and does not move his limbs as he should. In addition, certain signs will fairly soon become apparent; the child does not maintain its head posture, for example. A normal child when turned on its front will fairly soon be able to lift his head. Also when a normal child is held in the prone, that is turned from the supine position, he will lift his head and extend his arms and legs, whereas a child suffering from cerebral palsy will let both limbs and head hang passively. Even at this early stage, it may be noticed that the child is a poor feeder, has difficulty in sucking properly and that, when trying to feed, has problems with breathing. Clearly such children are liable to complications, not only of poor nutrition but also of respiratory infection and these must be dealt with. One should make it clear that many babies may display less than normal activity for a variety of causes, and the fact that a baby is less mobile than normal at this early stage does not necessarily mean that he has serious and profound brain damage. However, by the end of the second month the trained observer can notice that the child's motor development is subnormal. At this stage, a full physical examination may still be rather unrevealing in the sense that the normal parameters, for instance the head circumference, would be normal. The reflex activity of the limbs will not be abnormal, but it may be noticed that the two postural reflexes mentioned earlier, will not be present at this stage and that the child is not moving his limbs normally, is not paying attention to objects, e.g. following objects with his eyes or reacting to external stimuli in the normal way. At this stage, perhaps the most important thing is to make sure that fixed deformities do not occur and the child should have all his limbs put through a full range of passive movement.

Even at this stage, it may be noticed that the disability is confined to one side of the body, (hemiplegia) or confined to the legs, (paraplegia or diplegia) or that all four limbs may be affected (tetraplegia). It is perhaps worth noticing that a mild hemiplegia, (one arm and one leg being affected; the arm being affected worse than the leg) may easily be mistaken for a lesion of the brachial plexus, usually known as an Erb's palsy.

Although we do not know if there are any means of directly controlling the growth and development of the nervous system, we do know that if fixed deformities are allowed to occur and the limbs are in a poor posture, then undesirable reflex is developed which will further impair the child's function. In particular, disasters such as allowing the hips to become flexed and adducted, which may lead to dislocation of the hips, must be avoided. At the same time, prolonged splinting has a deleterious effect on the child's motor development and a regime of constant stretching, passive movements and assisted movements is usually the right course at this age. Cerebral palsy may be associated with other deformities such as club feet, thus if the child with club feet fails to sit up at the normal time, (at about six months) one should seriously suspect that there is an inherent disorder of the brain and nervous system. The failure of a child to start to stand and walk at a normal time, (at about a year old) in the absence of some gross orthopaedic deformity, such as dislocation of the hips, severe contracture of the knees, or severe foot deformity, might indicate cerebral palsy which is the commonest cause of delay in walking. It may or may not be associated with a certain degree of mental retardation.

Attitudes to management

Apart from preventing deformity and keeping all joints mobile, there are a variety of schools of thought about the best type of physiotherapy to give to children with cerebral palsy. One school of thought believes that the child should not be allowed to try to sit until it has good posture in a lying position, and should not be allowed to try to stand until it has good posture sitting, etc. This argument is based on evolution; the human organism has progressed from the fish to the amphibian to the quadriped to the biped stage. It believes that children with delayed nervous maturation should be forced to pass through the same evolutionary timetable. Another school of thought points out that as long as a child is supine it is not gaining adequate experience of the world or having adequate stimulus. It advocates that the child should be held in the upright position at the appropriate age even if this involves fairly complex special chairs holding the child's body and head in the erect position so that he can gain normal experience of the outside world. Equally, at a slightly later stage, there are those who believe that the child should be made to get on his feet when he has reached the age at which he normally would, and even if this necessitates giving him some form of external splinting or calipers or special standing or walking frame. It is felt that it is good for him to develop the feel of the ground, to develop postural reflexes in the joints and the soles of the feet. Obviously, the extent to which physiotherapy of this sort is given, must depend on the degree of the child's impairment. As however, the parents inevitably play a vital part in the management of a handicapped child, it is important that they should have some understanding of what is wrong. They should have everything explained to them at the earliest possible moment and should feel that everything possible is being done for their handicapped child. This applies, even if the child has a good deal of mental retardation and it is worth pointing out that even a limited walking ability enabling him to move to and from toilet, car or building to the wheelchair, with the minimum of help may make a great deal of difference to both child and his parents. Naturally, children who have motor disabilities of the arms may require special educational facilities and if they have locomotor disabilities of any severity can seldom attend an ordinary school. In addition to specific treatment of the child's motor problems, hearing aids, speech therapy, special educational methods and special social adjustments are all required (q.v.).

The child who has a disorder such as cerebral palsy must receive an amount of physical education comparable to the general schooling which is given to a normal child. The interruption of the pathways from brain to muscles may mean that the child does not develop the normal mechanisms of speech, seeing, hearing, limb and body control in walking, standing, running, writing, chewing and swallowing, or other vital activities. Training must be given by a team of specialists. This training will last throughout the formative years and the specialist team are best centred in one building so that schools for the complete education of the child from nursery to high school are usually the best answer (Figs. 9.2 a–d). These may be resident or non-resident, according to local needs. Such schools may be paid for and organized by local authorities but voluntary organizations are often the most vigorous in initiating and maintaining such schools. The staff of such specialist schools represent a synthesis of many diverse interests. There

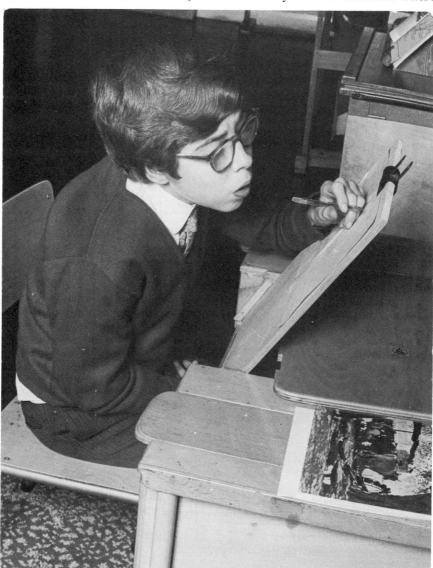

Fig. 9.2. (a) This handicapped pupil is using a specially designed board to help him write. (Figs. 9.2a–9.5 are reproduced courtesy of the Spastics Society).

are doctors of various specialities, nurses, physiotherapists, speech therapists, occupational therapists, social workers, teachers with special training for the education of the handicapped and many other staff members who form a large team with the main objective of giving the optimum education and medical care to the patient.

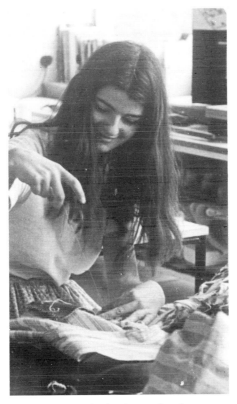

Fig. 9.2. (b) A cerebral palsy student learns to sew.

The management of patients with cerebral palsy

Patients with cerebral palsy have varying degrees of disability which range from those who have minor disabilities and who can live a relatively full and active life, to those who are so seriously handicapped mentally and physically that they can exist only with the totally dedicated care of parents or attendants within a house or institution. The term 'cerebral palsy' is sometimes called Little's disease, and is often classified as follows: spastic monoplegia, spastic hemiplegia, spastic paraplegia or spastic tetraplegia, rigidity, ataxia, paralysis and athetosis. The term spastic paralysis or cerebral

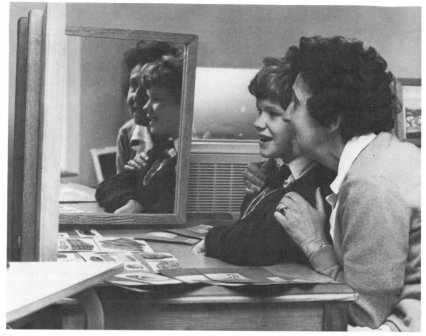

Fig. 9.2.   (c) A child using a mirror and pictoral aids in a speech therapy session.

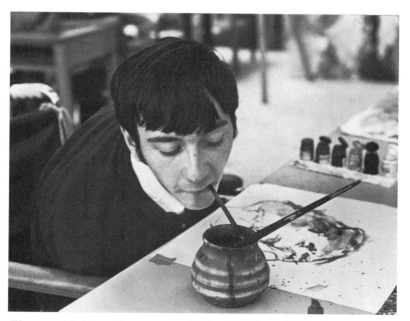

Fig. 9.2.   (d) A boy who cannot use his hands holds a paint brush in his mouth.

palsy, is an unfortunate one in that it lumps all patients together so that those who do not know, assume that all patients with this condition may be treated in the same way. Each cerebral palsy patient is different and requires adaptation of management to his particular needs. It is feasible that a mild cerebral palsy patient requires little or no medical, surgical or physiotherapy care.

Assessment

The most important aspect of the management is early diagnosis and comprehensive assessment of the whole problem. This assessment must commence as soon as it is recognized that all is not well with the child. The assessment team is made up as follows:

The paediatrician: He will be concerned with the accurate diagnosis of the disorder affecting the child and will lead the team and initiate activity by other members. He must eliminate other disorders which have similar symptoms and signs.

The educational psychologist: This worker is concerned with an accurate estimation of the degree of damage to the centres of the brain which relate to intelligence, memory, learning and aesthetic sense. He could be a major factor in placing the child in the best institution for his education. Brain damage, resulting in severe mental subnormality does occur and will greatly restrict any attempt at education. On the other hand the patient may possess a normal or high intelligence in a body which cannot see, hear or respond to its demands: this can be very frustrating to him.

The ophthalmologist: A problem, in the estimation of intelligence, is to know how good or bad the child's sight is. There may be a severe squint which gives the child an idiotic appearance which is not an indication of his true intelligence. The squint may be convergent—the eyes crossing, or divergent—the eyes separating, or concomitant—the squint alternating from eye to eye. In all cases there will be double vision and the child will deliberately retard the function of one eye and use a single eye for vision; this may be an eye which is pointed laterally or medially so that the child must poise the head in an odd position to use the single eye; thus the idiotic appearance is enhanced.

The ophthalmologist helps by re-aligning the direction of the vision of each eye by surgical means so that both eyes are pointed at the object in view.

Additionally spectacles may be provided to correct astigmatism. Thus the posture of the head is corrected and the interest of the child is stimulated by one form of management which gives remarkable results.

The otorhinolaryngologist : Again the ability to hear is related to learning. Speech and talking are learned by hearing and if the child cannot hear he cannot speak and may appear to be dumb. The ear, nose and throat consultant will arrange an estimation of the patient's level of hearing by audiometry. Any action which may improve the quality of hearing will also enhance the ability to learn and speak. Treatment may be surgical but most cerebral palsy patients with hearing problems are supplied with one or two powerful hearing appliances which enable communication by speech therapist, teacher, physiotherapist, doctor and parent. The result of improvement of hearing opens a whole new range of experiences for the deaf cerebral palsy patient.

The speech therapist : When sight and hearing are improved the speech therapist can do much to help the patient to communicate efficiently. She does this in many ways, all of which may be called 'communicating'.

The physiotherapist : Most cerebral palsy patients have involvement of the locomotor system. The physiotherapist will assist by assessing the weakness and strength of every muscle affected by the disability. The ability of every muscle can be recorded systematically and thus future physical therapy needs estimated. The chart records the strength in degrees from 0 to 5. Regular re-assessment will show which muscles require further development and which do not.

The occupational therapist : The occupational therapist is a major agent in assisting the patient to gain precious independence. The cerebral palsy patient is progressively trained to manage his activities of daily living, communication by writing or typing, and preparation for employment and earning a living if this is possible.

The Community Physician : Many of the agencies for the management of the cerebral palsy patient are under the control of the Community Physician. He may be the coordinating factor in relating the community services with hospital and educational needs of the patient. Transportation between home special school and hospital; ensuring that home circumstances are suitable for the management of the seriously disabled patient; supplying home helps; arranging advisers, community nursing services and many other aspects of the welfare of the patient.

Teaching staff : The cerebral palsy child's education usually commences earlier than that of the well child. This is because the services needed for his treatment are related to a special school.

A special school is one which is specially adapted to the needs of disabled children (Fig. 9.3). It is supervised by teaching staff with a head master or headmistress, rather than a doctor, physiotherapist, or nurse in

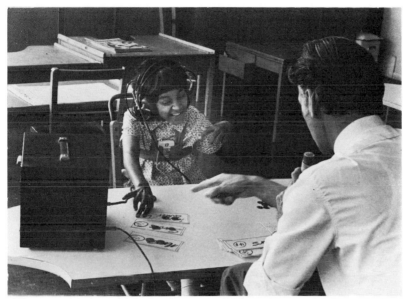

Fig. 9.3. (a) A multiple handicapped child receives special lessons using amplification of sound.

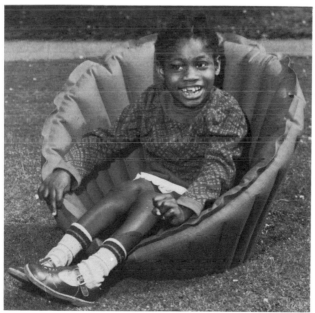

Fig. 9.3. (b) A specially designed chair.

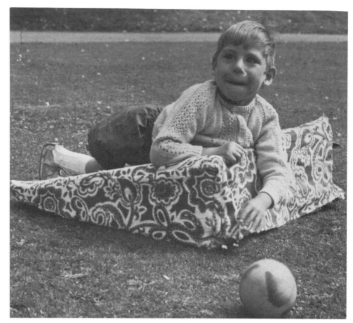

Fig. 9.3. (c) A wedged cushion to position a child with cerebral palsy.

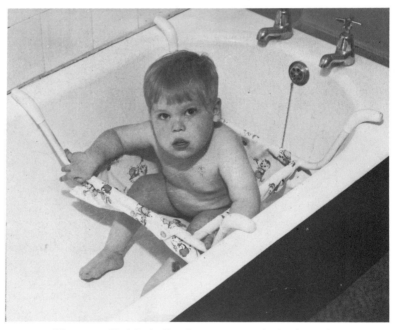

Fig. 9.3. (d) A bath sling for a young cerebral palsy patient.

charge. As full an educational programme as possible related to the treatment of the patient, is provided. Thus the special school has a comprehensive range of teaching units with accessory medical, nursing, physiotherapy and speech therapy facilities. The child's education, therefore, progresses but at different times of the day he will be taken from the classroom for treatment. The teachers assess, constantly, the ability of the patient and a full education is provided in primary, secondary, comprehensive and higher education schools and colleges.

The orthopaedic surgeon: The orthopaedic surgeon maintains a constant watch on the physical needs of the patient. He supports all the agencies already mentioned. He will advise on the provision of posture chairs, splints, calipers and other applinces (see Fig. 9.4), and will avoid and discourage any treatment which will seriously retard the education of the patient by prolonged or too frequent hospitalization. Many cerebral palsy

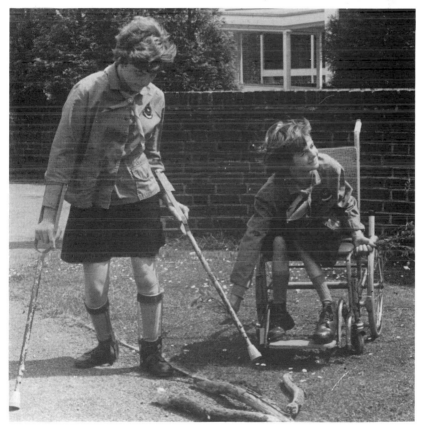

Fig. 9.4.   Calipers, crutches and a wheelchair used by cerebral palsy patients.

patients tend to manage a relatively full life despite their physical problems and it is often best to accept an ugly, awkward form of locomotion as long as the patient is able to move from place to place. It could be that surgical interference to improve posture or gait interferes with the patient's ability to walk and the wise surgeon often leaves minor deformities uncorrected.

The school nurse: Nursing is related to the degree of disability. The best attitude to any disabled patient is to encourage independence so that the patient can attend to his own total personal needs without help. Too much 'mothering' is, therfore, discouraged and training to manage self-feeding, lavatory routine and self-cleaning, washing and dressing is preferable. The nurse who eventually finds that she is 'redundant' in the care of a particular patient is to be congratulated in that the training of her charge has been effective. However, many cerebral palsy patients are so disabled that independence is not possible and they will always require total nursing care.

The principles of management

The child patient

As soon as an infant is diagnosed as a cerebral palsy patient treatment commences. Ideally it should be given each day and special arrangements may have to be made to locate the mother and baby near the treatment centre.

It is necessary to assist the development of the child in an attempt to create the same pattern and timing as far as a healthy child. This is done by repetitive movements which simulate the normal staged progression which should occur. If treatment commences soon enough, a considerable improvement may occur by the age of seven or eight. Training is needed to fit the child for coping with his environment. Thus sitting, standing, walking, climbing stairs, using the bathroom, manipulating knives and forks, handling coins, turning door handles and taps and all of the manipulating procedures which most people consider commonplace must be taught.

Much of the progress depends upon the will of the child and the encouragement of the helpers.

Equipment

Every child must be supplied with the furniture and items which are suited to his size and degree of disability.

CHAIRS

The height of the chair, the amount of support to the trunk and head which it must give, its stability, the safe positioning of the patient are all factors to be considered. Probably the best chair for the particular child is made by a parent handyman who is able to study the needs of his child and supply straps, pads and side-pieces to the guidance and specification of the physiotherapist and occupational therapist. Fixation in a chair must be limited to the times when it is essential for feeding or lessons. At other times the patient must be permitted to crawl and roll on the floor. The seated posture can cause flexion contractures of hips and a period of prone lying should be encouraged after sitting.

CALIPERS AND SPLINTS (see Fig. 9.5a)

When the knees and ankles are unstable it will be necessary to fit light-weight band-topped calipers to stabilize the legs and enable standing and walking. These are made of an alloy which is light in weight yet strong enough to tolerate the strains it will receive. Calipers must fit accurately and be replaced as they are outgrown. They can be fitted with screws and holes to enable them to increase in length but there comes a time when replacement is essential.

Careful observation of the limb in the splint is necessary. After removal of the caliper the skin of the whole leg must be examined for abrasions and compression through tightness. Daily washing of the limbs, a light dusting with talc, and a full range of passive movements to each joint must be carried out before application and after removal of the calipers. Careful maintenance of the splints is essential; checking for metal fatigue, washing away any soiling, saddle-soaping of leather; checking of footwear and splint-sockets in the heels of boots or shoes must be done daily.

It is often discovered, when the cerebral palsy team have admired the splints and calipers which they have provided, that the patient discards them as soon as he enters the door of his home. He then moves around, as well as he can, without them; perhaps he crawls or uses the family furniture to support himself around the house. It is always necessary to re-assess the need for a particular appliance. When it has served its function and is no longer of use it must be discarded or replaced. No equipment must be worn for the sake of appearances or because of what is 'in the book'.

WALKING AIDS (see Fig. 9.5b)

These vary from walking to sticks to tripods, quadripods, elbow crutches and axillary crutches. The supply of these is directly related to

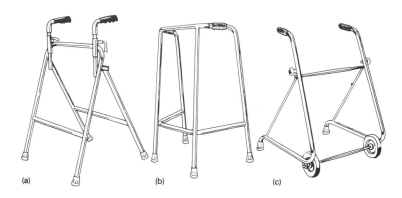

(a)   (b)   (c)

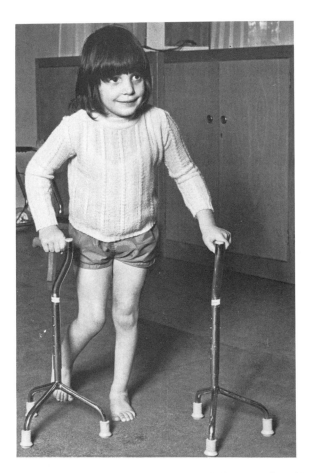

Fig. 9.5.   (a), (b) and (c) Walking aids. (d) Tripods being used to aid walking.

the degree of disability. If the child can manage without any so much the better.

WHEELCHAIRS (see Fig. 9.6)

The weight and strength of these will vary according to age, weight and degree of disability. Wheelchair living should only be necessary for the profoundly disabled cerebral palsy patient. It is preferable that if any form of walking is possible it is used.

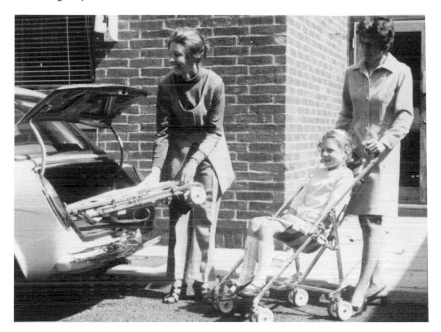

Fig. 9.6. A lightweight folding wheelchair for cerebral palsy children.

UPPER LIMB SPLINTAGE (see Fig. 9.7)

This is not usually desirable apart from hand-splints which may enable the child to place the hand in a more functional position for eating or writing. Sometimes a thumb splint which carries the thumb forwards into the opposing position has its uses in enabling the patient to grasp. It is always preferable that physiotherapy and occupational therapy increase the function of the upper limbs, rather than having them held in splints.

OTHER DEVICES

There are many other appliances for the use of the patient and some are shown in this section.

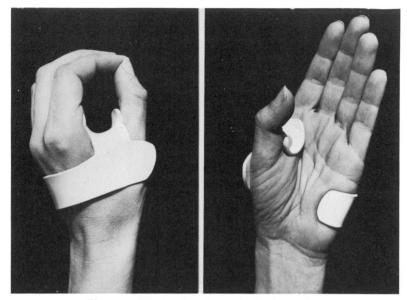

Fig. 9.7.   Hand splints for cerebral palsy patients.

Management of feeding

Speech and eating are related functions in that the muscles of mastication and speech are the same, and control of breathing and tongue are needed in both functions. Careful direction of eating will therefore assist the patient to improve speech.

Eating requires the ability to control:

1   the head, which must move forward to take the food from the implement.
2   the lips, tongue, soft palate, jaw and pharynx which must collect and swallow the food.
3   the larynx and epiglottis which must close off the respiratory passages.
4   the shoulder and elbow which elevate the hand to the level of the mouth.
5   the hand which must grasp the feeding implement.
6   the other hand which either supports and stabilizes the shoulder girdle as food is transferred from plate to mouth or holds the plate still as food is collected on the spoon.

Several factors must be considered in assisting the patient. These are:

1   The postural chair which must be properly related to the height of the table. Possibly the angle of the back of the chair can be varied for use during feeding.
2   The table. Often the normal household table is unsuitable and a special table is necessary.

Specially made tables should:

(a)   be of solid construction with a base wider than top.

(b)   have an easily cleaned surface which is cut out to fit closely to the shape of the trunk of the patient.

(c)   have devices for attaching the feeding dish to the surface.

(d)   have an overhead gantry to which slings may be attached as arm supports (see Fig. 9.8).

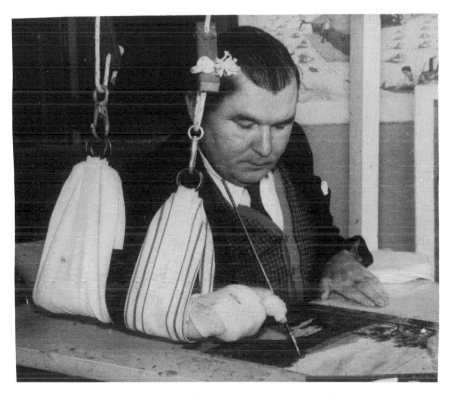

Fig. 9.8.   An overhead gantry for supporting limbs.

3   The clothing. A waterproof smock is an advantage.

4   The food. This must be 'spoonable' but not tedious. The child will quickly resent tasteless slops and such food is not necessary. It is possible to supply a good balanced diet of items which can be either collected on a spoon or grasped.

5   The implements for eating. The variety of these is wide (see Fig. 9.9) and occupational therapists are usually experts in devising spoons with special handles which are angled to meet the personal needs of each patient.

Additionally the dish may be provided with a special rim against which the food may be held.

It is essential that the family of the patient are fully instructed in the method of feeding and the reasons for such careful instruction.

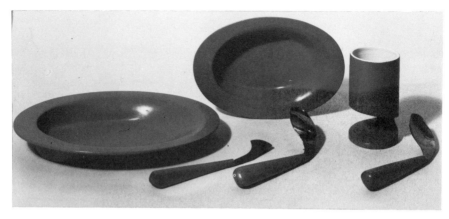

Fig. 9.9. Implements for assisted feeding.

10 : Basal Ganglia and Cerebellar Conditions

Relevant anatomy and physiology

THE BASAL GANGLIA

These are collections or clusters of nerve cells; they are situated in the base of each cerebral hemisphere and they are often referred to as the basal ganglia or basal nuclei. They are close to the stem of the brain (see Fig. 10.1).

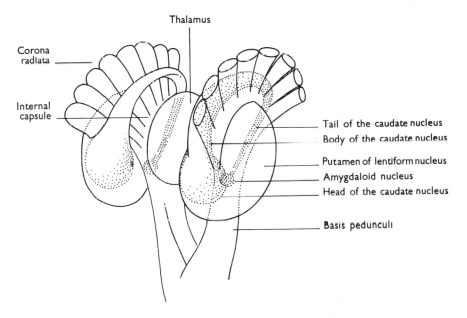

Fig. 10.1. The situation of the basal ganglia.

The basal ganglia comprise:

1   the thalamus; 2   the corpus striatum; 3   the lentiform nucleus; 4   the caudate nucleus; 5   the amygdaloid nucleus; 6   the calustrum.

The capsule (see pyramidal tract) runs between them. These are all areas which serve important functions, with responsibility for specific activities concerned with muscular coordination. There are interconnecting pathways between them and also connecting fibres to the cerebellum and cerebrum and anterior horn cells or lower motor neurone nuclei.

The cerebellum

This occupies the posterior lower area of the vault of the skull underneath a transverse diaphragm or membrane called the tentorium cerebelli. It is oval in shape with a central constriction and is flat on its upper surface (see Fig. 10.2).

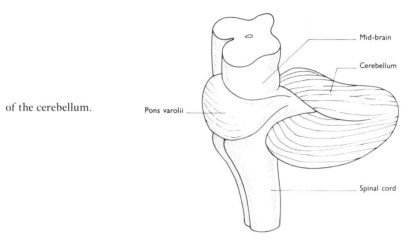

of the cerebellum.

Pons varolii

Mid-brain

Cerebellum

Spinal cord

An important structure is the connecting bundles of pathways which communicate with the cerebrum, the medulla oblongata and the pons Varolii and the anterior horn cells.

THE FUNCTIONS OF THE BASAL GANGLIA AND CEREBELLUM

Impulses from:
1   the motor areas of cerebrum, from
2   the balancing organs (semicircular canals) of the ear, and from
3   the muscles of the neck and trunk enter the cerebellum via the connecting bundles of fibres.

This area of the brain is, therefore, an important area of communication with other parts of the brain and body. They are particularly concerned with balance and equilibrium; the tone of muscles; the coordination of muscle contraction and relaxation; the ability to place a limb accurately, that is, put the hand or foot precisely where it is desired to place it. Co-ordination of the hand or foot, spatially, when an object is to be touched or grasped; steadiness of movement; absence of tremor; and fine precise movements such as writing, embroidery or ballet dancing or walking along a line all depend on the physiological integrity of these centres.

Disorders of this area will cause dysfunction in all or many of these activities so that imbalance, spasticity, failure to relax, flaccidity, tremor of movement, inability to position a limb precisely or do fine work, or to walk steadily and elegantly are all manifestations of disorders of these parts of the brain.

DISORDERS OF THE CEREBELLUM AND BASAL GANGLIA

So far, we considered lesions of the cerebral cortex and internal capsule, lesions of the long spinal tracts and lesions of the peripheral nerves. There are also centres within the nervous system, which play an important part in the control and coordination of muscular movement. These centres comprise anatomically, the basal ganglia and the cerebellum with their spinal and cortical connections.

The exact functions of these centres are best understood when one observes the disorders of function which result from lesions in these sites.

Cerebellar lesions

Lesions of the cerebellum produce nystagmus, ataxia, hypotonia, intention tremor and post pointing or overshooting the target: in animals, unilateral lesions produce postural deformities such as spinal curvatures. We might describe the cerebello-spinal system as an essential part of the finely controlled system by which the antagonistic muscles increase their activity towards the end of a movement, until finally their tension equals the tension of the prime movers and the limb is held steady in a new position. The cerebellum may be affected in certain hereditary disorders such as Friedreich's ataxia, in disseminated sclerosis, by injury, tumour or arteriosclerotic disease.

Basal ganglia lesions

Lesions of the basal ganglia produce excessive rigidity hypokinesia and constant coarse tremor. The patient has a mask-like facies, a typical, rapid shuffling gait and a constant 'pill-rolling' hand tremor. He has great difficulty in initiating any movement, e.g. he or she cannot start walking, but if rocked from side to side, can start walking, but may be unable to stop. In addition, the patient has dysarthria and may suffer from oculogyric crises. The condition may occur as a sequel to encephalitis lethargica, as the result of the effects of certain drugs, e.g. phenothiazone, or of manganese poisoning or as a result of cerebral arteriosclerosis.

Treatment

There is usually no specific treatment which can reverse the disease process and restore normal function. Treatment is therefore mainly palliative. In addition to certain drugs (see below) remedial exercises have some value but above all helping the patient to adapt his mode of life is of great importance. Therefore, physiotherapy and the drugs, atropine, belladonna, hyoscine and a variety of synthetic drugs such as benzhexol, all act primarily by blocking the muscarinic effects of acetylcholine. Alternatively levadopa may be used to boost the defective inhibitory effect of lack of dopamine. It must be pointed out, however, that all these drugs, and levadopa in particular, may have undesirable side effects which can make them unsuitable for any given patient.

External appliances are not usually of much help nor do operations on the limbs play any part in treatment. At all costs, the patient should be kept active and external splints usually have a harmful effect causing pressure sores and making the limb stiffer and less useful. Even after a fracture, the minimum of external splinting should be used; as unfortunately, the constant repetitive muscular contractions also make internal fixation harder and less effective. In selected patients operations on the basal ganglia may relieve rigidity and diminish tremor. It is probably in this direction that we can look for future advances but at the moment such operations are often unpredictable and while they may relieve spasticity and tremor they often lead to loss of power and paresis and may further impair function.

Parkinsonism (Fig. 10.3 a and b)

Parkinsonism is a syndrome. This means that there are several symptoms and signs which indicate the presence of the disease. In this case tremor, rigidity of muscles and clumsiness of movement are the main problems. But related to this are the many personal functional problems of the patient, such as the inability to stay quite still, to hold the pen to write in the normal manner, to put food into the mouth using the usual implements, to keep the tongue and head still, to walk without a slow cumbersome gait. For the person who has led an active life, with use of all his faculties, to be affected in this manner in the later years is frustrating and depressing.

A wide range of therapeutic management has been tried and in recent years stereotactic surgery to create a small circumscribed lesion in the brain

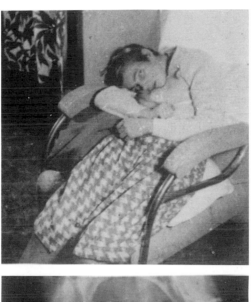

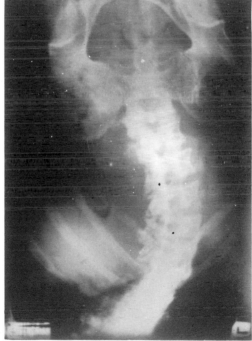

Fig. 10.3. (a) Parkinsonism. Severe flexion to the right with dominance of rigidity on the right side. (b) Radiograph of the spine of the patient.

was extensively tried. Most forms of treatment have side effects, however, which are often worse then the initial problem. For example, stereotactic surgery relieved the tremor but also reduced the power of the limbs so that the patient had weakness or even paralysis.

Levadopa and Parkinsonism

It was discovered by neurophysiologists that dopamine, which is a catecholamine losely related to adrenaline and noradrenaline, was a neuro-transmitter. Dopamine is a substance released in the normal brain to cause transmission of impulses from one neurone to another.

In 1960 it was then discovered that dopamine was reduced in secretion in patients suffering from Parkinsonism. Logically, by supplying dopamine in pharmacotherapeutic form it is possible to correct the depleted secretion of dopamine, but dopamine alone cannot cross from bloodstream to brain.

The same neurophysiologists then tried levadopa which is capable of crossing from blood to brain where it is changed to dopamine by an enzyme. This has caused dramatic improvements in *some* patients who relate their experiences of discarding the wheelchairs and crutches after needing these for several years.

However, the drug is not suitable for all patients and there is no known way of predicting the response of particular patients. There are also side effects to levadopa including giddiness due to a fall in blood pressure, personality changes, confusion, gastric distress, increased pulse rate and involuntary unpredictable movements of the limbs and face.

Huntington's chorea
(Chronic progressive chorea; hereditary chorea, familial chorea)

This is an inherited disease which is not sex-linked and may be trans-mitted by either the father or the mother to their children when either parent has inherited it from one of their parents. One of the misfortunes of this condition is that symptoms and signs do not usually appear until the fourth or fifth decade of life (sometimes later) by which time the patient may have already raised a family some of whose members will already be affected.

GENETIC COUNCELLING

It is now possible to recognize a prospective hereditary chorea patient before the symptoms and signs appear. When there is a family history of such disorders advice must be sought either before marriage and certainly before starting a family.

SYMPTOMS AND SIGNS

Huntington's chorea is a disorder which produces two main effects upon the body; choreiform movements and mental deterioration. Thus, there may be mental dementia associated with chorea.

CHOREA

This is a symptom of many neurological disorders when the basal ganglia and cerebellum are affected. It consists of unexpected, involuntary, jerky movements of the limbs and face and body which embarrass the patient because they make him conspicuous.

The movements may be unilateral or bilateral; that is, the arm and leg and face on one side only may produce the choreiform movements or both sides may demonstrate the erratic uncontrolled movements. The patient is usually in a constant state of fidgitiness or twitching even when sitting or lying down.

MENTAL DETERIORATION AND DEMENTIA

This may occur before the chorea is demonstrated or both effects of the disease may be seen together. At first there is a decline in intellectual efficiency. There may be depression with suicidal tendencies and with severe irritability and personality changes. Often these patients are admitted to psychiatric hospitals for treatment before the condition is diagnosed. There are severe emotional and other difficulties.

The symptoms and signs are infinitely variable from one patient to another. Progress of the disease is rapid in some patients and in others it may be some years before the symptoms become troublesome. Others may be only mildly affected throughout their lifetime. There is no reliable way of telling which form of the disease will occur in a particular patient. Because one member of a family is affected it does not necessarily follow that others will be too.

INHERITANCE

Every patient with Huntington's chorea carries the responsible gene. The gene is the unit of inheritance which is responsible for all of our inherited characteristics such as eye colour, facial contours, intelligence, stature, blood group and sex (see Fig. 10.4).

In an inherited disease, such as Huntington's chorea, the normal gene has been altered or is deficient in its ability to cause certain essential chemical

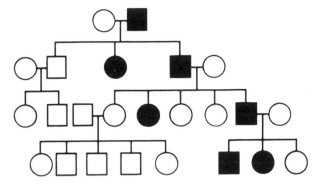

Fig. 10.4. Normal and abnormal genes showing autosomal dominant inheritance.

substances to by synthesized so that the chemistry of the affected body is altered.

This eventually produces the symptoms and signs of the disease if the patient lives long enough. He or she is also liable to pass on the disordered gene to his children who in turn will pass on the gene to his grandchildren. Thus the disease can affect many generations of a family and it is possible to trace and recognize the condition in the ancestors and kin of current patients.

The principles of management of the patient with locomotor dysfunction

Disturbances of the locomotor system are common to many diseases, most of them neurological. Although treatment must deal with the present and the immediate future the long-term problems must be considered.

As there is a probability of progressive deterioration a tactful balance between optimism and realism must be attempted. The intelligence and mental condition of the patient must always be considered and the skill of the nurse or other health worker in applying the correct and acceptable approach to the patient and his immediate relatives is an essential part of management. Sometimes there are remissions when symptoms disappear and the patient improves and is filled with hope that he is cured. Substantial improvement in the early stages may result in severe depression and disappointment when this does not continue. There may be marked variations in performance so that one day the patient is walking or speaking or writing and the next is unable to achieve any objective. Many of these variations are related to fatigue, elation, depression or any of the emotions or factors encountered in everyday life. The patient should be aided to work and establish a pattern of living which avoids fatigue or depression. Management is related to each phase or stage of the disease as it manifests itself. In the early stages the symptoms may be so slight that the patient is unaware of them unless comments are made by others.

Acceptance by relatives

The neurological patient often has a gait, mannerisms and peculiarities which are symptoms of his condition; these may make him unattractive to his family and in the community. It is not easy to accept a person who may be chairbound, mentally subnormal, socially unacceptable and requiring a great deal of repetitive intimate care for the remainder of life. Such a low state is found only in a small proportion of these patients, however, and many require little assistance, and certainly less than these notes indicate. When possible it is better for the patient to return to his own environment; he can experience loneliness and isolation just as a healthy patient and no institution can replace the warmth of acceptance in the family circle.

The nursing staff should work towards the preparation of his relatives for the return of the patient to his home whilst he is still under treatment in hospital. Graduated return may be possible—encouraging the family to take the patient home in the knowledge that if the problems are too great, return to hospital is easily achieved for further rehabilitation. If this fails, admission to an institution which is properly staffed and equipped is better than endangering the health of a spouse or parent in the attempt to manage an impossible situation.

Public attitudes

Understanding from those who are not family members is necessary, but not always available. They may assume that the patient is under the influence of alcohol or drugs and make unkind comments to the patient or the relatives. Modification of community attitudes by propaganda is necessary.

Training to achieve standing and walking

When the patient can stand and possibly walk—no matter how badly— a degree of independence has been achieved which gives optimism to both the patient and his relatives. He who can walk can reach the bathroom! The ability to progress to the bathroom means release from the misery of soiled beds, bedpans, urinals and commodes which must be emptied and cleaned, for both patient and attendant. The physiotherapy staff work to this end from the day of admission of the patient to hospital. Muscles which are not paralysed must be prevented from wasting; methods of rising from a bed or chair must be taught; the best possible gait in the light of the disability is learned. Tripods and stands, walking machines, splints and crutches all have their place in the process of achieving some form of locomotion (see Fig. 10.5)—no matter how slow and ungainly.

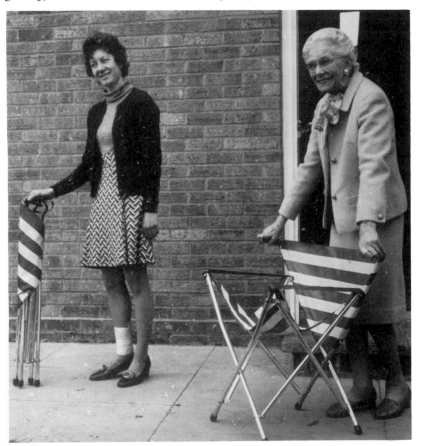

Fig. 10.5. An example of a walking aid.

Independence in feeding and the personal toilet

Probably the most time-consuming aspect of patient care is that of feeding. In hospitals it is a worry for an administrator to find sufficient people who have the time to sit by the bedside of helpless patients feeding them with small portions of food until the meal is consumed. It is often a greater problem in a family circle where the members must go to work or school or where patient care depends upon a single individual with limited time for many chores.

If the patient can learn to transfer food from crockery to mouth—even crudely and slowly—it relieves the hard-pressed family and makes the patient feel a degree less useless and futile. The same applies to washing, shaving, using the lavatory and dressing.

There are many aids which have been devised to assist the patient (see Chapter 12) in achieving a return of independence in these habitual tasks. The occupational therapy staff and social workers can advise on the method of obtaining such aids, which are often custom-made to suit the individual.

Retraining for employment

It is not an easy matter to find employment for a person with a severe disability. Legislation exists in many countries which ensures that the large firms employ a small percentage of the physically handicapped population on their staff. The employer is more likely to employ a lightly disabled person to fill his quota than one who is slow and requires special concessions and considerations. Legislation usually does not apply in this respect to small firms with a few employees.

There are some state-assisted factories and voluntary organizations which help to find employment for the physically handicapped. The social worker assists by introducing the patient to the disablement resettlement officer whose task is to find suitable employment for disabled persons. Often some form of home employment is all that is possible in the light of the disability, and frequently there is nothing.

A positive approach to general health

Even though the patient has a severe neurological disorder which is untreatable, much can be done to ensure that no secondary conditions contribute to his problems. A full assessment of the patient, therefore, is made so that treatment can be arranged for any associated condition. Upper respiratory tract infections and other septic foci are cleared with antibiotic therapy. The eyes are tested and spectacles supplied if necessary. If hearing can be improved with a hearing aid this is done.

The problems of the patient's family

Any of the conditions discussed in this chapter severely affect the whole family. The same constant whole day care given to patients in hospital must be applied by fewer people in the home. Perhaps a solitary spouse must care for the patient as well as completely run the household; buying food and other essentials, cleaning and cooking. Often a husband is unable to go to work because there is no one else to care for his severely disabled wife and so there is also severe financial distress. Older children may need to discontinue schooling to assist in running the home.

All of this merits a full range of state aid in practical social and financial terms. There must be an adequate funding of the family by the state to prevent hardships for the patient or relatives. Help from expert advisers is equally as important as practical help from domestic workers and the medical officer of health and community nursing service must be totally involved in ensuring that all help is given.

Probably the gravest problem is that of social isolation and loneliness caused by rejection by neighbours or extra family relatives. Caring for a seriously disabled person can mean long periods of confinement to the home with no relief by visits to cinemas, theatres or social clubs. A holiday away from home is often impossible either for financial reasons or because there is no hotel or boarding house which can cope with the many problems of the patient. Amenities in most societies require fitness and the ability to deal with stairs and fast transport; the disabled are not catered for or the minimum is provided. Even shopping has become a process requiring youth and fitness; supermarkets are not places for wheelchairs or crutches.

Many philanthropic organizations exist to help but often they are distant from the patients home or too heavily loaded with work for others. It is possible for most patients with severe disability to go on an annual holiday to a specialized centre for their management but often this is the only relief in a year of limited living.

11 : Infections of the Central Nervous System

Relevant anatomy and physiology

The central nervous system, because it is composed of delicate and vulnerable tissue, is protected from tauma by a bony case, skull and spine, a thick outer and two thin inner membranes, dura mater, the cerebrospinal fluid and a fluid suspension medium. Another form of protection is also essential; defence again infection.

The normal defence mechanisms, which are provided for all other body tissues, also operate within the central nervous system. Because of an excellent blood supply to the meninges, the ventricles, and the canals with a circulating fluid (cerebrospinal fluid) the defence mechanisms against infective changes on the other hand are effective; the nerve cells are very vulnerable and unlike most cells are not capable of dividing and regenerating, so infections of the central nervous system are potentially very damaging.

THE BONY CASE

The whole central nervous system (the brain and spinal cord) is encased in a bony box, and a thick membrane—the theca, which has controlled exits and entrances. The arteries enter the cranium, via openings in the base of the vault of the skull, an almost direct route from the left ventricle of the heart. The veins, similarly, return to the heart by an almost direct route. The only other entrances and exits in the skull and theca are the openings through which the cranial and spinal nerves pass.

Thus the bony case and theca protect the central nervous system by isolating it. The rate of flow of blood into the theca is controlled by the carotid sinus which acts as a governor. Reflexes from the carotid sinus alter the diameter of the carotid vessels and the heart rate and blood pressure.

The meninges

Among the many general functions of the meninges, in relation to the nervous tissue, one is to contribute to the anti-infective barrier. The meninges additionally have further functions specific to each meningeal layer and the structure of each is directly related to its function:

THE DURA MATER

The most superficial of the three meningeal layers is the dura mater. This is a tough fibrous membranous lining attached to the interior of the cranium and the neural canal of the vertebral column. It serves to contain the cerebrospinal fluid and nervous tissue within a waterproof and micro-organism-proof sac (see Fig. 11.1).

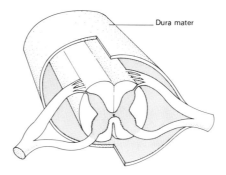
Dura mater

Fig. 11.1.   The dura mater as a protective covering.

THE ARACHNOID MATER

This fine web-like layer is loosely laid inside the dura mater. It has a highly vascular structure with many blood vessels and capillaries contributing to it. Additionally there are many lymph nodes which have a direct function in combating infection in the central nervous system.

THE PIA MATER

This forms a sheath to invest the brain and spinal cord and thus retain the central nervous system within a neat package. The layer again contributes to the anti-infective barrier which protects the nervous tissue it contains. Penetration of the surface of the brain by microorganisms, which could cause a brain abscess, is made more difficult by the pia mater. The arachnoid and pia mater have relatively little mechanical strength and only play a minor part in protecting the central nervous system from injury but are very important in their ability to react to infections. However, after the infection has been overcome they may remain thick fibrous and adherent. Their nature has been changed by the infection and thus may lead to permanent serious sequelae.

CEREBROSPINAL FLUID

The many functions of this fluid are not yet fully understood. The support of the central nervous system within a fluid medium, protecting it from injury during running and jumping or when a severe blow is applied to the head or back of the trunk, are obvious functions. It is also involved in the transmission of nutrition to the nervous tissue within the theca.

A function, which is particularly relevant to this chapter is to protect the contents of the theca from and to combat infection which has gained entrance via the circulating blood (haemotogenous infection) or by penetrating wounds such as would be caused by a lumbar puncture or cisternal puncture needle or as the result of trauma (direct infection).

Cerebrospinal fluid is not just a watery filtrate derived from the blood. Its composition is related to the function which it must perform. Suspended in a high water content are proteins, amino acids, glycerol, glucose, chlorides and gases. In health few white cells (lymphocytes—about 5 per cubic millilitre) are found. In the presence of infection, however, there is a large increase of lymphocytes and in acute infections polymorphonuclear cells also appear in the cerebrospinal fluid to meet and deal with the invading microorganisms. When specimens of fluid are collected by lumbar puncture in the diagnosis of intrathecal infection the lympocytic count is usually found to be high and the presence of polymorphonuclear cells indicates an inflammatory reaction.

PHAGOCYTOSIS

The central nervous system has an excellent blood supply which is carefully monitored by special mechanisms such as the carotid sinus. In the presence of infection there is an increase in the blood supply and a rapid and massive increase of the leucocytes in the blood. When infection invades any part of the body, the leucocytes isolate, kill and remove the offending organisms which enter the central nervous system.

LYMPHATIC DRAINAGE

Debris and micro-organisms from the central nervous system are removed from the theca by the lymphatic route, as in any tissue. Within the arachnoid mater are lymphatic vessels and nodes which collect and destroy invading micro-organisms.

Infections of the central nervous system

Infections of the central nervous system arise from three main sources:
1   there may be blood-borne infection, particularly meningitis secondary to cerebral abscesses which are often secondary to a lung abscess.

2   penetrating wounds, either stab wounds, gunshot wounds, compound fractures or surgical intervention, may all be followed by infection
3   infection where there is a fistulous connection between the subarachnoid space and the surface of the body either following injury, or operation or occasionally as a result of a congenital abnormality by which infection may travel into the central nervous system.

MENINGITIS

Clinically there are four main types of infection of the central nervous system. There is first of all meningitis which will cause irritation of the meninges, ophisthotonos, pain, photophobia, impairment of cerebration and pyrexia. If left untreated meningitis will ultimately cause the death of the patient. Nowadays with the use of antibiotics it is usually possible to control the infection but the patient may be left with a varying amount of disability, usually disorders of movement similar to other upper motor neurone lesions as well as varying degrees of cerebral impairment, deafness and blindness.

Occasionally, some years after an attack of meningitis, where there have been adhesions, cysts develop which may spread and enlarge and mimic a cerebral or spinal tumour.

EXTRADURAL ABSCESS

Extradural abscesses may occur either in the brain or in the spinal cord. Their importance in the spinal cord is that they are usually secondary to osteomyelitis of the vertebrae. Their presenting symptoms is first of all, very acute backache and the patient may be misdiagnosed as being hysterical. Their great importance is that if rapid treatment is not instituted there will quickly be thrombosis of the spinal vessels leading to complete and irreversible paraplegia.

CEREBRAL ABSCESS

Cerebral abscess which as explained, may follow a penetrating wound or middle ear infection. Usually in addition to the systematic evidence of toxaemia and pyrexia, there will be neurological evidence of an expanding space-occupying lesion which if left untreated will lead to disorders of consciousness, drowsiness, paralysis, blindness, vertigo, deafness, and ocular paralysis.

SPINAL CORD ABSCESS

Lastly, abscesses of the spinal cord itself and of these the chronic abscess of tuberculous infection, in the tuberculoma, used to be most common; it can mimic very closely a spinal tumour. Treatment in the initial stages is beyond the scope of this book, but of course the residual lesions which are usually of an upper motor neurone type, that is with spastic paralysis of a different degree, will require treatment on the lines indicated elsewhere (Chapter 6).

Antimicrobial chemotherapy for infections of the central nervous system

Following the introduction of antibiotics and chemotherapy in the management of infections of the central nervous system the whole pattern of treatment has changed. Whereas with pre-chemotherapy regimes, little could be done to save the life of or prevent serious permanent disability to, the patient with meningitis or encephalitis, nowadays swift positive and specific treatment, the relevant chemotherapeutic or antibiotic therapy will arrest the course of the infection before destruction of nervous tissue has occurred or become significant.

There are problems in the use of this form of therapy on the patient. Reference to the applied anatomy and physiology section of this chapter (pages 241 to 243) will indicate that the central nervous system is situated within a special compartment of the body to protect it from trauma and infection. Not only does the antimicrobial barrier serve to keep out infection; it also serves to impede the transmission of some drugs and other substances from the bloodstream to parts of the central nervous system.

Drugs, which are introduced into the body via the oral or parenteral route (intravenously for example) will take a longer period of time to reach the inside of the theca and may be too late to prevent damage to nerve tissue by the infection. The medical officer in charge of the patient will therefore probably choose to introduce the relevant antimicrobial substance directly into the theca via a hollow needle. This should result in an instant local effect within the central nervous system.

Choice of a specific antibiotic

This is most important in the management of this form of infection. Again there are problems here. A blood sample may not contain the organisms which are affecting the central nervous system and a specimen of cerebrospinal fluid obtained by lumbar puncture may be needed for identification of the causative organism. Delay, due to the time lapse which is needed to culture the organism, before the antibiotic is introduced is dangerous. A broad spectrum antimicrobial therapy is commenced until the specific therapy can be started when the micro-organism has been correctly identified; an example of the therapy used in the urgent undiagnosed case would be chloramphenicol with sulphonamide. When the pathological department has had time to report on the cerebrospinal fluid specimen submitted for culture, the therapy used will depend upon the organism present. Examples of specific antibiotics and chemotherapy used in the management of meningitus would be:

MENINGOCOCCAL:
Penicillin (or ampicillin) with sulphonamide.

PNEUMOCOCCAL
Penicillin (or ampicillin) with sulphonamide in large doses.

HAEMOPHYLLIS INFLUENZAE
Ampicillin with sulphonamide.

STAPHYLOCOCCAL:
According to sensitivity.

ENTEROBACTERIAL:
According to sensitivity.

TUBERCULOSIS:
Streptomycin with Izonicotinichydrazid (INH) and Para-amino-salycilic-acid (PAS).

Common symptoms and signs of severe acute infections of the central nervous system

Because the central nervous system affects all other organs and areas of the body the presence of infective changes will result in unusual and profound effects. The reactions to such infections may be classified as those which are general and those which are specific to infections of the central nervous system.

General reactions

I   TEMPERATURE CHANGES
In high fever the recorded temperature will show a sharp swing up-

wards. This will result in severe fluid loss by perspiration and probable dehydration of the whole body. The effects of this will be:

(a)   Diminutia of all glandular secretions except sweating. Dry mouth and eyes may leads to ulceration and serious secondary complications.

(b)   Reduced urinary output.

(c)   Constipation.

(d)   Toxaemia.

(e)   Loss of appetite.

2   CARDIO-VASCULAR CHANGES

As the normal reaction to infective changes and leucocytosis there is an increased flow of blood to the affected part. There is a general increase in bloodflow to the skin to dissipate heat. The respiratory system also requires an extra blood supply. This results in:

(a)   An increased heart rate and pulse.

(b)   The volume of the pulse is also raised.

(c)   There may be flushing of the skin.

3   RESPIRATORY CHANGES

The respiratory rate is increased and there may be irregularity of respirations with a foul-smelling breath.

4   MENTAL CONFUSION

The rise in temperature and the toxins produced by the micro-organisms will result in severe mental disturbance which is additional to the local problems in meningoencephalitis.

5   RIGORS

Specific reactions

The following symptoms and signs may appear in varying degrees of severity related to the areas of the central nervous system affected. The micro-organism causing the infection and the degree of infection are also related factors:

Severe headache

Stiffness of the neck and back

Paraesthesia

Somnolence, then stupor and disorientation and eventually coma

In children, convulsions may occur

Muscle spasm and paralysis of the spastic type
Tremors
Photophobia
Opisthotonos
Positive Kernig's sign

Recovery depends on the amount of nervous tissue destroyed by the infection. Time is all important in the management of the central nervous system infections. Early diagnosis should precede immediate use of the specific antibiotic and chemotherapy. The longer the delay the worse the resultant permanent brain or spinal cord damage.

The management of the patient with acute infection of the central nervous system

The patient with severe toxaemia due to infection will be abnormal in all respects. Mental confusion, pain, dehydration, severe hyperpyrexia and perspiration contribute to an illness which requires good nursing and careful medical management.

The patient is best nursed in a quiet room away from traffic noises and unnecessary movement. The brain and spinal cord are in an irritable state and any jarring by sound, sight or movement may result in nervous spasms (or convulsions in an infant). Opisthotonos is a state which exists when all the extensor muscles of the back, neck and thighs are in spasm and the patient's back is arched. Excess bright light or jolting of the bed may bring on this severely painful state. It must be reported at once so that the relevant muscle relaxants may be considered.

A firm bed without head pillows is best in the acute stage but the reader is referred to the section about paralysis in poliomyelitis on page 252. Clothing and coverings should be minimal and if the room is warm enough light coverings should be adequate.

Observations and diagnostic measures

The nursing measures related to chart and observation must be comprehensive as they are an essential guide to progress. The frequency of the observations depend upon medical instructions. They include:

1   Temperature, pulse rate and volume and respiration rate and volume.
2   Blood pressure
3   Eye pupil state
4   Response to questions or calling the patient's name

5   Estimation of degrees of spasm or paralysis
6   Reflexes which are present or absent
7   Rigors
8   Fluid balance

Additionally regular estimation of the physiological chemistry of the patient is made by the pathologist who will require

1   Lumbar puncture to collect specimens of cerebrospinal fluid,
2   Venupuncture to collect specimens of blood for electrolyte analysis, leucocyte estimate, bacterial culture,
3   Urine specimens to indicate the chemical output of the patient.

Drugs and pharmacology

As a result of these specimens specific solutions for intravenous parenteral infusion will be prepared to correct any biochemical abnormalities. This solution for the antibiotics and chemotherapy. During lumbar-puncture the opportunity will also be taken to introduce the relevant antibiotic.

The severe headaches and muscle spasm will be relieved by the use of sedative, analgesic and muscle relaxant drugs.

Nutrition and diet therapy

During an acute infection the main dietary need is for fluids which must be supplied in large quantities, if necessary, by intravenous infusion. These contribute greatly to the treatment of the patient. Even if the patient can swallow, any food which requires gastro-digestive effort will probably be vomited. When the pyrexia has passed, greater effort to maintain a good nutritional standards can be made. Most fluid intake will be by the parenteral route.

Surgical intervention

When a brain abscess exists in a site which is accessible to the surgeon, an operation may be performed to release pus and debris. The patient's head must be shaved and full pre-operative preparation made. If the abscess can be localized the pus can be drawn out by aspiration with a wide-bore needle and a suitable antibiotic instilled into the cavity.

Keeping the patient's airway clear

The patient is vulnerable to obstruction of the air passages by inhaling vomitus, saliva or blood. This is a disaster which must be avoided and constant observation is essential.

The dentures are removed from the mouth of the patient and stored for the duration of the illness. The foot of the bed is elevated to cause secretion to gravitate away from the air passages and towards the mouth from where they can be aspirated by the use of suction apparatus. The position of the patient is important. This is in the semi-prone position (see Fig. 11.2).

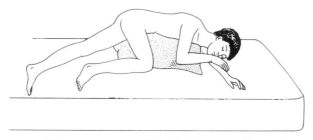

Fig. 11.2.   The semi-prone position for the unconscious patient.

When severe unconsciousness ensues, the surgeon may decide that a tracheostomy and insertion of a cuffed tracheostomy tube are desirable. This permits much more precise control of the air passages in the prevention of obstruction of the airway. It has, however, the disadvantage that infection of a long continued tracheostomy is almost inevitable and in hospitals colonization of tracheostomies by antibiotic resistant organisms is very common.

Permanent brain damage

The danger of severe localized or generalized infection or trauma of the central nervous system is residual permanent destruction of the nervous tissue. Depending upon which segment of the brain is affected the patient will have varying forms of disability. There may be mental subnormality with loss of memory, aesthetic sense or response to the environment; speech may be affected; hearing may be slightly or severely affected; sight, either vision or the ability to focus on precise points may be affected; the basal ganglia or cerebellum is affected, will result in loss of coordination of muscles and choreiform movement or ataxia or paralysis may occur.

All of these require special management, mainly to enable the patient to live within the limits of his disability.

Acute anterior poliomyelitis

Poliomyelitis is an infection caused by one of three types of virus. This micro-organism usually gains entry to the body via the gastrointestinal tract. After a period of incubation the virus attacks the central nervous system at any level of the spinal cord. As a result of this infection the spinal cord will undergo the inflammatory changes much as any other tissue of the body.

At first there is an increase in the blood supply in the area of infection; then the nervous tissue becomes inflamed, oedematous and swollen. As a result, certain neurones lose their function and paralysis of the muscles served by that segment of the spinal cord will result. The amount of paralysis suffered by the patient is directly related to the quantity of nervous tissue affected. It varies from a disastrous complete paralysis affecting the whole trunk and all the limbs, to a minor weakness of individual muscles or no paralysis at all. Later, this inflammation resolves. There may be no after effects of the inflammation that is complete healing of the nervous tissue, in which case there will be no permanent residual paralysis; or the neurones may be destroyed or scarred with permanent disability. It must be emphasized, however, that only one-fifth of all patients affected by acute anterior poliomyelitis have paralysis.

Many nations have a vaccination programme against this disease which immunizes whole populations in childhood so that the major epidemics which were common in the past no longer occur. As there are still nations without an immunization scheme, however, poliomyelitis must still be considered a hazard to health. Epidemics nowadays are more likely to occur in areas where public health standards are low.

THE PATTERN OF ACUTE ANTERIOR POLIOMYELITIS

This disease may be considered as having five distinct stages:

1 Incubation
2 Onset
3 Greatest paralysis
4 Recovery
5 Residual paralysis

1 *The stage of incubation.* This lasts approximately fourteen days. It is the time when the virus has entered the body and is multiplying; the nervous tissue provides a good culture medium for this type of virus. The patient will have no symptoms or signs. It is considered by some that the amount of destruction of nervous tissue is related to the activity of the patient in this stage; the more sedentary person will suffer less disability than the active athletic individual.

2 *The stage of onset*. Lasting forty-eight hours, this stage gives symptoms and signs which are similar to an attack of influenza. These may be mild, a coryza with headache and malaise, or more severe including pains in muscles with stiffness of the neck, spine or limbs.

One problem during an epidemic of acute anterior poliomyelitis is to know which disease is affecting the patient—influenza or poliomyelitis? As many patients with poliomyelitis recover at this stage and possibly have not called for medical help, it is difficult to know. We know that many adults have had subclinical attacks of poliomyelitis. The danger is that the patient remains a carrier for a long period after a subclinical attack and may provide a reservoir of micro-organisms to maintain the epidemic in a community.

The majority of patients with mild infections recover after this stage. During the latter part of this phase the patient may have symptoms and signs of meningeal irritation.

3 *The stage of greatest paralysis*. During this eight-week period the patient has paralysis directly related to the amount of nervous tissue involved. The anterior horn cells of the spinal cord are swollen and oedematous and unable to function in the affected area. If a large segment of the cord is affected, there will be major paralysis affecting a large number of muscles, on occasions the whole body from the neck downwards and including the respiratory mechanisms may be paralysed. If only a small number of neurones are affected, the patient may have a paralysis of one or a few skeletal muscles.

An important principle of the management at this stage is to realize that it is the nervous tissue and not the muscular system which is infected.

In the care of the patient's muscular system there are four objectives:
1 The prevention of contraction of muscles.
2 The prevention of stretching of muscles.
3 The maintenance of a full range of movements in all the joints
4 The prevention of deformities.

If the thoracic muscles are affected, the maintenance of adequate ventilation of the lungs is another requirement.

4 *The stage of recovery*. This can extend for a period of up to two years. There is a slow resolution of the inflammatory changes in the spinal cord. Motor neurone (anterior horn cells) which have been temporarily affected, but not destroyed, recover their function. As the nerve pathways which serve the affected skeletal muscles regain their function, so do the muscles.

The degree of recovery is variable from one patient to another. Some gain a great amount of function in their affected limbs and muscles; some hardly any or none at all.

An important attitude in this stage of management is to avoid over-optimism in the patient. There is hope that complete recovery will occur, but it is best that the patient learns to adapt to his existing disability and lead as full a life as he can. If full recovery does happen, this is a reason for rejoicing but foolish optimism must not retard progression to useful and happy living with the disability.

At first recovery is rapid; later the rate of improvement becomes less. After one year a big change is unlikely; after two years the condition is static.

5 *The stage of residual paralysis.* (Fig. 11.3). After the two years, it must be accepted that any paralysis remaining is permanent. The surgeon may decide to aid the limited function of the patient by the transplantation of

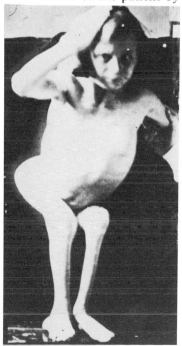

Fig. 11.3. A patient with severe paralysis as the result of poliomyelitis.

muscles, elongation of tendons, tenotomies, arthrodesis of joints, neurectomy and any other form of surgical intervention which will assist the locomotion, posture or usage of the patient's limbs or body.

The management of the patient with acute anterior poliomyelitis

At all stages this requires a comprehensive team of workers representing most facets of patient care.

During the stages of onset and maximum paralysis the patient may require intensive care, particularly if the respiratory mechanism is affected. Intermittent positive pressure ventilation, parenteral nutrition or tube feeding, a consistent two-hourly turning routine and special bladder and bowel management may be needed for the survival of the patient. Such care is carried out in special hospital units and is beyong the scope of this book.

Up to six weeks from the start of the illness the patient's faeces contain the micro-organism of poliomyelitis and he is therefore infectious to others. His attendants must be adequately immunized against the infection and the patient nursed in isolation.

Relevant nursing and physiotherapy and management

The orthopaedic and physiotherapy team must have access to the patient at the commencement of his illness, particularly if there is paralysis present. The orthopaedic management of the patient may be classified into the following phases:

(a)   Ensuring that during the stage of greatest paralysis, deformity is avoided and that muscles and joints are maintained in the optimum condition for later rehabilitation.

(b)   Later careful assessment of the degree of pralysis present, in particular muscles, classification of the strength of the affected muscle and prevention of the deterioration of that function until recovery.

(c)   Providing planned and logical rehabilitation during the stage of recovery to give the patient optimal improvement of function.

(d)   Supplying adequate means for the patient to cope with any residual paralysis. This may mean surgical intervention, such as muscle transplantation, or the provision of appliances such as calipers and wheelchairs.

(e)   Retraining the patient for daily living and earning a means of livelihood when a disability is premanent.

All of this requires adequate communication between each member of the team and the patient. The most effective course of action to aid the recovery of any patient can only be decided upon at a conference of all the health workers involved. Thus a meeting of the surgeon, physical medicine consultant, nurse, physiotherapist, occupational therapist, medical social workers and the disablement resettlement officer must be convened at relevant stages in the progression of the patient towards recovery. An ideal would be to involve the patient in the meeting, but if this is not possible he must be made aware of the decision taken at the meeting and his cooperation sought.

Prevention of deformity during the acute stage

The whole body of the patient is nursed in the optimum position of rest. This means that the patient is supported in a posture which ensures that no joint is held constantly in a position which will overstretch any muscle or group of muscles.

The nursing positions used are similar to those for the care of patients who have spinal injuries or paraplegia or tetraplegia, as described in Chapter 5.

The principles of positioning are:

1   The head and spine are supported in the normal anatomical position, without distortion.

2   The shoulders are arranged with the arms either in abduction or flexion, depending upon the position in which the patient has been placed.

3   The elbows are adjusted into about 45 degrees of flexion.

4   The wrists are supported in an extended position with the hands arranged around cylinders which are about 10 cm in diameter.

5   The hips are arranged in partial abduction and partial flexion. Extreme lateral rotation is prevented by the use of supporting pillows.

6   The knees are flexed.

7   The feet are maintained at right angles by the use of firm pads.

It is most important that no part of the patient is maintained constantly and relentlessly in one fixed position so that a contraction requiring attention develops. The patient's position is altered at two-hourly intervals and on turning, the position of the shoulders, elbows, hips and knees is passively varied for him.

If a muscle group has weakness or paralysis there is a danger that the opposing muscle group will force the joint or limb into deformity. For example, the action of the posterior muscles of the forearm, supplied by the radial nerve, is to pull the wrist and fingers backwards into extension; if the lesion in the spinal cord affects the radial nerve, the posterior muscles of the forearm will be paralysed and the powerful anterior muscles will tend to pull the wrist forwards into a flexed position—this is known as a 'drop wrist'.

It may be necessary in these circumstances, to supply a plaster shell or splint to prevent deformity and to maintain the joint in an overcorrected position. This shell is removed at regular intervals so as to move the joint passively through its full range of movement before the splint is reapplied. The objective is that when and if recovery of the nerve occurs, the muscles and joints will have normal function. The splints supplied must be light in weight and should support, not fix, the affected part.

Management during the stage of recovery

As part of progression towards the stage of recovery, the physiotherapist makes an estimation of the power of function of individual muscles. Various tests are used; some of these tests can accurately assess the function of a muscle so that its power can be recorded and improvement indicated at successive testings. Electromyography is used to indicate muscle activity; when a muscle tissue contracts, electrical potentials develop the electromyograph amplifies these potentials and records them graphically. Power in a muscle is recorded by a figure between nought and five; nought indicates that there is no power and five indicates full power.

When it is established that power has returned to an affected muscle, or that a weak muscle is gaining strength, the physiotherapist commences re-education of the muscle until maximum recovery has been reached.

It is essential to know which muscles are functioning and which are not before deciding when the patient may progress from the horizontal position first to sitting and then to standing. For example, if the muscles which normally support the vertebral column are weak on one side (muscle imbalance) sitting upright without adequate support to the spinal column could result in a postural deformity such as scoliosis.

Relevant management for the stage of residual paralysis

If sufficient time has elapsed and no recovery has occurred in certain muscles or muscle groups, it must be accepted that the patient is left with a permanent disability. The patient must learn to enjoy as full a life as he can within the range of that disability.

12 : Practical Aids and Equipment for the Paralysed Patient

Mankind is characterized by its ability to use tools and utensils. People who are paralysed need a greater variety of tools, splints, aids and appliances in their everyday lives more than the unparalysed. The range of equipment which is commercially available is enormous and there are large lucrative industries and firms totally dedicated to producing, modifying and improving the devices used by the invalid and disabled person.

Needless to say much of this equipment is expensive to buy. Often this is because each item is custom made and this requires hours of work on the part of a craftsman. Another reason for high cost is that many of the items are under patent in another part of the world and the patentee has the sole rights on the production and sale of an item.

However, many of the items of most practical use to a disabled patient can be made out of less costly materials by a 'do-it-yourself' handyman. There are often simple easily made items which are best fitted and shaped for the individual.

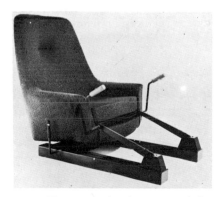 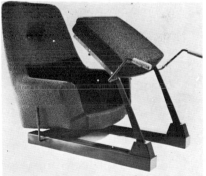

Fig. 12.1. An ejector type chair to enable a patient to rise from sitting.

Not unexpectedly many of the best aids have been designed by paralysed patients for themselves. In so far as most aids require some effort and adaptation before maximum utility is obtained it is natural that patients often

257

make the greatest use of their own 'brain-children'. Also standard appliances often require slight modification and adjustments to suit the individual patient.

The place of the 'handyman' in the life of a paralysed person is important. Much comfort can be given to patients in their homes by the adaptation of furniture which can only be correctly fitted by 'trial and error'; in other words modifying and re-modifying after fitting and comment by the user of the item.

To raise or lower?

Commonplace household furniture can be modified in many ways to the personal convenience of a paralysed or disabled person. Heights are all important. Probably the greatest need of the patient which can be satisfied is correct adjustment of his personal furniture to the level which suits him. This is often critical to the patient and a few centimetres difference in the height of a chair may make it possible for him to stand from sitting or sit from standing or to feed himself without help from others.

Adjustable and temporary or fixed and permanent?

There are problems to be considered about this question. Adjustable and temporary devices too often are weak and unreliable. Adjustability is convenient when several people with different heights, sizes and needs are using equipment. But the furniture may be at the wrong height when the patient who needs the item most wishes to use it. Additionally the patient must have faith in the reliability of his equipment and although an adjustable item may be reliable, the patient may not trust it and awkward movements may become unsafe when he tries to modify his poor abilities to meet the lack of trust in the equipment. Therefore the strong, solid and obviously reliable furniture is often preferable. Every physiotherapist knows that really solid rigid parallel bars are necessary to give confidence to a nervous paralysed patient who is learning to walk again. Although wobbly bars do not actually collapse and let the patient fall the feeling of insecurity is often adverse to the patient's balance and confidence.

Correct heights

Beds, chairs, tables, working surfaces, sink units, baths, lavatory pans, bidets, cistern levers, taps or faucets, sticks for walking, crutches, quadripods, tripods, steps and stairs, and even boards on which to stand must often be adjusted to the exact heights and levels which are needed by that particular parient. If a foot cannot be lifted far from the ground because of paralysis the bound edge of a thick carpet can constitute an obstruction to mobility and often be a hazard. If a lavatory seat is too low it cannot be used.

Within a household, it may be that most items are arranged to the height needed by the disabled mobile patient and accepted by the other members of the family or else only the furniture most used by the paralysed person is permanently arranged to meet his needs. There are many factors relevant to this decision but they mainly centre upon the attitudes of the family to the patient or the patient to his disability; many would prefer that the less obvious the problems the better; too much invalid-type impedimenta can only advertise the presence of the patient's ailment.

Correct weights

Lightweight, flimsy furniture is often least desirable. However, if the patient must lift and carry the item it must be as light as possible (see Fig. 12.2). These factors therefore help to decide the materials which must

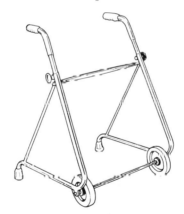

Fig. 12.2.   A lightweight walking aid.

be used. If an item is to remain permanently in one position and the person is to lean heavily on it to sit from standing or lie down from sitting or reverse these movements then heavy fixed pieces of furniture are preferable and iron, steel and hardwood are preferable materials. If the patient must wear or transport the equipment then lightweight alloys or balsa wood are essential to avoid stress or fatigue. There must, however, always be considerations of strength related to lightness. Items which break in use and or are costly to replace often endanger the life or health of the patient. There are biomechanical engineers, metallurgists and craftsmen who specialize in such knowledge, and have developed excellent purpose-made invalid furniture (see Fig. 12.3).

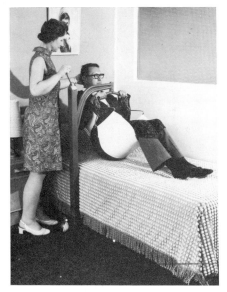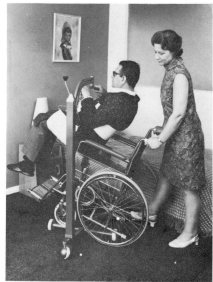

Fig. 12.3. (a–b) A wheeled hoist for lifting and lowering the invalid.

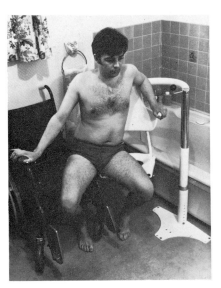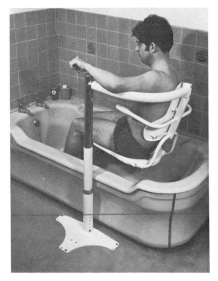

Fig. 12.4. A hoist designed to lower the invalid into the bathtub.

Buckles, clips, fasteners, studs and straps

In no other situation is the choice of the correct fastening for the particular need more important than in clothes, splints and appliances for a paralysed person. The problems are:

1   Poor or absent tone in the adjacent muscles.
2   Lack of firmness in skin.
3   Absence of sensation from skin to central nervous system so that the patient is unaware that a strap or fastening is hurting.

So careful choice of fixation of any equipment is necessary. If leather straps and buckels, or metal clips are used there must always be a protective layer of material between the skin and fastening. If the tissues of a paralysed patient are damaged it may mean prolonged treatment and restriction of any activities.

Probably the happiest invention for any disabled person has been the Velcro strap (see Fig. 12.5). This has a construction which makes it fasten strongly when two surfaces meet and thus there is no need for buckles or clips which might injure skin and other tissues.

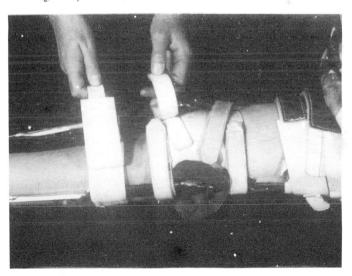

Fig. 12.5.   Velcro straps.

When strength is essential then leather straps and buckles or press studs may be the only choice.

The criterion in choice of a strap of other fastening must be the independence of the patient related to his ability to fasten the strap himself, unassisted. Dependence on others must be avoided if possible.

There are situations where a strap fastening cannot be used and a crepe bandage is the only means of fixation possible.

Aids to mobility

1 Aids to walking

FUNCTIONS

(a) To receive the weight of the body and thus avoid it being applied to an injured or painful limb. Crutches (elbow or axillary) are examples of this type (see Fig. 12.6).

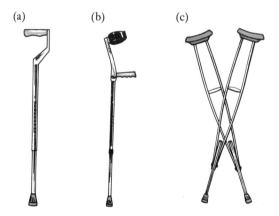

(a) (b) (c)

Fig. 12.6. (a) Lightweight walking stick; (b) lightweight elbow crutches fitted with swivel arm band and fully adjustable; (c) axillary crutches.

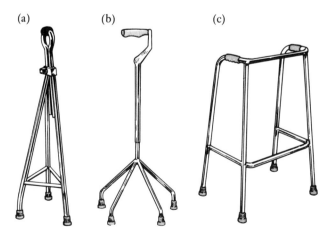

(a) (b) (c)

Fig. 12.7. Balancing aids to walking (a) adjustable tripod aid; (b) lightweight quadruped adjustable walking aid; (c) walking frame.

(b)   As a balancing device when there is loss of coordination of limbs and the feet cannot be placed precisely. Such problems exist in multiple sclerosis and tabes dorsalis among many other neurological conditions. A stick or tripod can serve as a third support to avoid topling over (see Fig. 12.7).

(c)   As an indication of handicap. An obvious example of this would be the white stick of the partially-sighted person but other disabled people may wish to indicate to others that they have physical problems.

The selection of the most suitable walking aid for each patient is important as is the estimation of the correct height and weight. Such decision-making will often require discussion between the physiotherapist, occupational therapist and doctor. The correct training in the use of the device is also essential. A patient with severe problems and impairment of communication will often require prolonged instruction and supervision.

One criterion for the use of any walking aid is safety. It is essential to know that the ferrules are of the non-slip type and worn-out ferrules must be replaced immediately. Related to this is the need for selection of suitable footwear. Sloppy, loose or slippery shoes must not be used. Many modifications to footwear are available including height alterations, and variations in angles to meet particular problems.

Wheelchairs

When all forms of walking are impossible, the only recourse is to wheelchair mobility. If the patient is well endowed with money or financial support from the state or other sources he will find a wide range of wheelchairs available to him. The wheelchair is selected according to the needs of the patient related: (a) to the disability, and (b) to the uses the wheelchair must serve for the patient who has achieved a wide spectrum of independence.

Wheelchairs may be:

(a)   *Heavily padded and supportive.* When extensive paralysis and sensory impairment exists, a heavily-padded chair is the only one feasible. If the patient's trunk is paralysed and his spinal and other muscles will not support him in the upright posture he must be equipped with a chair with a tall back to it to hold him in a correct posture.

(b)   *Electrically driven.* A motorized wheelchair with special joy stick controls can be supplied for a patient who cannot move a chair by pulling on the wheels or who has severely restricted movements. They require constant maintenance to ensure that the electrical battery is charged daily and serviced.

(c)   *Lightweight and highly mobile* (Fig. 12.8). These have similarities to a

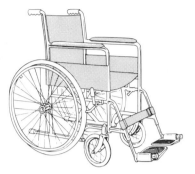

Fig. 12.8.   A lightweight alloy wheelchair.

racing bicycle. They are made of lightweight alloys which require little effort on the part of the patient to move them. A patient whose disability affects only his legs and whose trunk, upper limbs and neck are unaffected

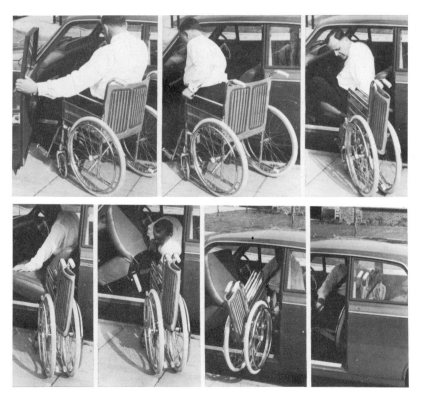

Fig. 12.9.   A lightweight alloy wheelchair and a specially designed car allow this paraplegic patient independence and mobility.

can achieve a high speed in such a chair. On a suitable surface he can often cover as much ground as the unparalysed person in less time.

(d) *Folding, collapsible and lightweight* (see Fig. 12.9). These are suited to the paraplegic car driver who wishes to move out of his chair and into his car and then lift the chair on to the rear seat of his car.

No matter which chair is used by the patient it is essential that he fully understands the dangers of remaining in the chair without relieving the weight of his trunk from his buttocks and pelvis at regular short intervals (see Fig. 5.16).

Automobile transport

Many patients with lower limb paralysis can drive a car. The preference is usually for a car which is similar to any other vehicle rather than one which carries the stigma of disability. Most conventional vehicles can be so modified. When severe disability exists, however, there may be no alternative but to supply an invalid car, and to use specially designed slings (see Fig. 12.10).

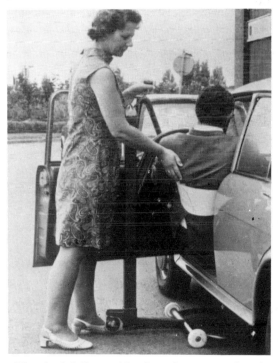

Fig. 12.10.   The wheeled sling enables the patient to move from house or wheel-chair to car.

13 : Social Services and the Care and Rehabilitation of the Disabled

To a variable but increasing extent in the last twenty-five years the ultimate central responsibility for social services and welfare in most countries has been carried by the government. The government usually controls its social and health services through a special department of health and social services. Such central control, however, is too remote from the people who need the services and these must be administered by a local authority.

The local authority responsible for the provision of help for the disabled may be the same as that which is in control of all the other essential services in an area; housing, land control, water supplies, sewage systems, refuse disposal, ambulance services, road making, police, schools, electrical and gas supplies, burial grounds, cremation and many other aspects of local government which are necessary for the welfare of any community. If provision of help for the aged, paralysed and physically handicapped, mentally ill or subnormal is included in this long list it may be that these will have a low priority, inevitably but unfortunately, since increases in local taxation (rates) are never popular, this is often the case. There are many countries where provision for any of these categories is minimal or does not exist. Others have an excellent record of caring for those in need of help and have every reason to be proud of their achievements. Generally such provisions are related either to the wealth or poverty of the community or to its form of government.

The present organization of welfare in the United Kingdom is as follows:

The director of social services and coordination

Within a local governing authority there is a social services committee which has an executive officer in charge of the services known as the Director of Social Services. His main qualification for his post is a wide knowledge of the national legislation relevant to the disabled and handicapped, the financial provisions for their care, the source of funds for giving help, the voluntary bodies, national and local and the functions of the many staff of the local authority related to the care and rehabilitation of the disabled. Part of his or her function may be to call on the help of such unlikely bodies as the engineering departments of the local government, for instance, when adaptation of housing or provision of specially-modified public lavatories for the use of the disabled are required. The overall purpose of such a Director of Social Services is therefore to coordinate the many aspects of the care of the disabled which exist in a community, which might, without properly directed organization, dissipate their funds and efforts to less purpose than when coordination exists. The director must be a person with a deep sense of the needs of individuals who have physical problems. He must be ready to be unconventional and imaginative in the application of laws and regulations related to his work; there is no place for a bureaucrat who works strictly 'to the book' or remains in his office.

Local voluntary bodies

In addition to the funds and services available from government sources, there exists in most countries of the world, a large number of local voluntary bodies who are working for the handicapped. Examples include organizations for the blind and deaf, spastics society, councils for the disabled, a multiple sclerosis society, organizations for the care of the aged, the crippled children, the mentally handicapped. In addition there are auxiliary nursing and first aid associations, and ex-military, naval, air force, police or fire brigade benevolent associations. These are organized and run by people with altruistic motives towards their fellow men. This motivation may be religious or emotional but there is no doubt that much help and support for the disabled may be given when such groups of people are well organized and vigorous. Many local government bodies give financial help to support these organizations.

Medical and nursing services related to the social services

Any disabled person, no matter what form his disability takes, whether physical, mental ophthalmic, auditory, or due to senility, needs care. Once the patient is recognized as having a problem there should be a coordinated effort by all members of the health and welfare services team. Continuous and consistent effort should see the person through to full rehabilitation or support him in the optimum state of finance and comfort which can be provided in an institution or in the normal home environment.

There must be no division into fragments of the care of a patient. Care begins when the general practitioner attends the patient at home prior to sending him to hospital. It is continued at the door of the hospital as the patient is admitted, and when the patient goes to convalesce. The final aid is when the patient is attempting to make the best of his life and problems who no further progress towards his physical recovery can be made.

'Total patient care' should see the patient through from beginning to end of his illness with assessment of the care he will require. There should be a smooth transition from stage to stage with all aspects of health care; medical, dental, physiotherapeutic, nursing, occupational therapeutic and dietetic. Social rehabilitation, financial assistance, home adaptation and provision of special equipment for his disability, employment resettlement and any other relevant needs should be supplied and coordinated without delay or duplication of effort. There is a need for fusion between general community, medical and nursing services; hospital-based services and social workers in hospital and local authority. Thus, community health services should have full access to the hospital and the patients, and the hospital-based services should leave the hospital premises to oversee the patient in his home when this contributes to his recovery.

The help needed by the disabled person

It is not possible to generalize in classifying the help needed by a person with a disability. Each must be seen as an individual and the aid given must be modified to the particular person. There is no place for firm, fixed and inflexible rules laid down by governmental decree; it is better that broad principles, supported by good legislation and financial cover, exist and that field workers, with imagination, freedom from restriction and a desire to give comprehensive help are permitted to do so. The help needed is infinitely variable from person to person. There are those with severe handicaps who will require little help and those with lesser disability who need much aid. Probably the greatest need is freedom from financial stress in a competitive society where the capable and clever can live in full luxury but the weak and ailing are often deprived.

The help needed will vary according to:
(a)   the age of the patient,
(b)   the attitudes of his or her next of kin,
(c)   the numbers of relatives or good neighbours available,
(d)   the psychological state of the patient, whether cheerful and optimistic or morose and pessimistic,

(e)   the nature of the handicap,
(f)   the geographical environment, whether town or country, crowded or sparsely inhabited,
(g)   the voluntary help organizations in the locality of the home,
(h)   the financial state of the individual.

No matter what circumstances exist, the objective for all those who aid the patient must be a return to normality or as near to this as is possible. Institutionalization is the least desirable state but is, unfortunately, often the line of least resistance, for those with responsibility. If the attitude and living conditions of the family and community can be modified so that the patient can be accepted back into familiar surroundings this is preferable. Often there is strong initial resistance to this but once the idea is accepted and the necessary support given, it is found to be preferable.

'Help, not pity', should be the motivating theme for anyone concerned with the disabled and the help must always be positive and effective, overcoming all obstacles while being resilient and unconventional. It is, however, important that outside help should also encourage the patient to do as much as possible for himself. Overprovision may undermine a patient's morale and make him too dependent. Every patient—however old or infirm should be encouraged to do as much for himself as possible   even if 'doing it yourself' takes longer. It is important that patients feel that there is a reason for going on trying.

The social worker

The social worker is a person with wide terms of reference related to different people with varying problems. For the purposes of this book we refer to the disablement social worker with particular interest in the problems of the handicapped.

The social worker is trained particularly to assess the problems of the patient, record the activities needed to resolve them and seek and arrange the help necessary for each individual. Perhaps the most important function of the social worker is coordination in arranging that every form of feasible help is directed towards the person who needs it. Such functions as arranging for a blind person to learn Braille or to receive a radio set or tape recorder; for a deaf person to have a hearing aid; a paralysed person to have help in cleaning the home or to be equipped with all the necessary aids for the paralysed; for a handicapped child to have full schooling with necessary transport to achieve this; for all sources of money to be taped for the impoverished; for youth to visit and talk with the lonely aged; for the religious to have spiritual comfort; and the demented to have supervision. In fact, ideally the social worker should know how to supply any needs. He or she is often only limited by the amount of imagination shown by those who can give help.

Disablement resettlement officer

A disablement resettlement officer is probably best defined as a social worker who acts as a liaison between industry or commerce and the handicapped person who needs work. Employment for any person with a disability is a problem. Finding employment for people with some disabilities is often a more serious problem than for others. Patients with a psychiatric history or epilepsy are usually the hardest to place but all patients with residual or progressive disabilities require much effort to arrange placement.

Some countries have legislation which requires that firms which employ a given number of workers must take a percentage of disabled workers (in the U.K. this is 4 per cent). However, it is often difficult to define the degree of disability of a handicapped person. To stay within the law, an employer may take on a complete quota of persons with minor disability to exclude those with serious problems such as paraplegia.

To employ persons with serious handicaps may require some modifications to the premises of the factory, shop or office. An obvious problem is that a wheelchair worker must be on the ground floor (or near a special elevator) and have access to modified washrooms, lavatories and perhaps cafeterias. Why should an employer provide these facilities when there is an ample supply of fit skilled workers?

Often, however, employers are fiercely altruistic. Once the needs of a person are defined and there has been complete and honest communication of the problem by the disablement resettlement officer the employer will try hard to create the environment and circumstances in which the physically handicapped person can work.

Probably the most serious problem in arranging a place of employment for a disabled person is reliability. It can be exasperating for any employer of labour to have to cope with an employee who is consistently unpunctual or absent without warning. Often the problems of people with handicaps are unpredictable; a bad night spent without sleep because of pain, gastric distress or incontinence can mean the need for much more time in preparing for work next morning; if the central heating has gone off in the night the patient may be unable to start the long tedious process of dressing and toilet before heating has been arranged.

It is often the case that once employment has been found, the disabled employee ensures that he retains his job by being overpunctual and reliable; probably more than the fit healthy workers who surround him. There are a few employers who would prefer certain work to be done by disabled persons because of their consistent reliability and high workload. There are certain types of monotonous repetitive work which are specially suitable for the mentally subnormal and some employers prefer such workers.

Sheltered workshops

Probably the greatest source of employment for disabled people is the factory provided by a government especially for the training and employment of those who are severely handicapped. This movement was started by Sir Robert Jones in the United Kingdom when he was Inspector of Military Orthopaedics to the British Allied Armies during the 1914–1918 Great War. These are centres with complete adaptation of the premises to the needs of the worker in a wheelchair, on crutches or unable to follow a conventional pattern of behaviour at work. Such sheltered workshops of course cannot be supplied in sufficient numbers to meet the needs of every unemployed disabled person.

The unemployable disabled

There are many disabled who cannot be given employment because they are unable to pursue any sort of normal life beyond the boundaries of their own dwelling. It is possible for some such patients to have employment within their homes related to their intelligence and manual dexterity. An obvious example would be television programme monitoring by a tetraplegic person or communicating by telephone on behalf of an organization which communicates to a mailing list in this fashion. Often work, such as finishing the packaging of their products, may be given out to people working at home.

Activities of daily living

An important aspect of improving the lot of the physically handicapped is an assessment of their activities of daily living. This is usually most effectively carried out by an occupational therapist whose training includes this ability. She will estimate all that the patient can achieve towards independence for activity at home. She will classify the patient's independent

activities into areas such as:
(a)   *Bed activities*
Ability to turn to right or left
Sit up from lying
Sit erect from bed
Stand up from bed
Reach and use the commode
(b)   *Personal care*
Wash: 1 Face
        2 Arms and hands
        3 Chest to waist
        4 Below waist
Shave
Clean teeth
Groom hair
Manage on toilet
Self-care after toilet
Manage lever on cistern of toilet
Turn taps on or off
Get into or out of bath
(c)   *Consumption of food*
Use fork, knife and spoon
Use spoon only
Drinking from vessel
Using a drinking straw
(d)   *Dressing*
Fastening clips
Fastening buttons
Fastening Velcro straps
Put on socks or trousers
Pull garments over head
Put on shoes
Manage prosthetics
(e)   *Wheelchair or other mobility*
Propel forward or backward
Turn right or left
Use in various situations
Relate toilet and wheelchair
Relate bath and wheelchair
Move from wheelchair to bed or toilet and vice versa

(f) *Laundry*
Ability to wash small items
Ability to use washing machine
Peg out clothes
(g) *Kitchen*
Control of gas taps or electric switches
Loan and unload oven
Manage electric kettle
Open tins of food or cellophane packages
Peel vegetables
Cut bread
Boil milk or eggs or vegetables
Heat prepared foods
and many other categories and divisions related to the particular patient.
From the report of the occupational therapist the support needed by the
patient will be assessed.

Training centres may be provided to assist the patient to improve performance in these activities. Various gadgets may be supplied to assist the
patient to manage activities which are impossible or difficult without them
(see Chapter 11).

Transportation

The means of moving from place to place determines our way of life.
The owner of a car and sufficient money to buy petrol to use it has a far
wider choice of dwellings, work and recreation than the person who has
no car or cannot afford to run it. Although the fit person without a car
cannot be so selective in his abode at least he can use his legs or public
transport to achieve a reasonable way of life. To the disabled the means of
transport may be the difference between a miserable, lonely way of life or
a full active one with the capacity to earn. Yet often the handicapped person
cannot afford a vehicle because his earning capacity is so limited. It is
therefore necessary for the state to consider that the provision of such
transport is as essential for the disabled person as an artificial limb is for
an amputee. The vehicle supplied must be one which can be managed by a
person who has severe limitations yet which does not stigmatize him. Provision of transport must also include consideration of supplying a garage
access to his house and maintenance for the vehicle. When the patient is
unable to manage to drive himself then he must be driven. The local
authority may supply special vehicles with hydraulic lift for collecting
patients in wheelchairs for outings or essential visits.

Relief from monotony

Probably the most serious problem for the patient and his attendants is boredom. Confinement to one room with the restrictions of a disability may mean a sameness of living which goes on day after day, year by year without relief. The patient becomes detached from the realities of living, isolated and lonely and may eventually demonstrate psychiatric distress. This problem also reflects upon the relatives of the patient; maintaining a consistent programme of care for a person living the whole of the day 'year in year out' restricts the way of life of the attendants to the same level as the patient.

Therefore, some form of relief from monotony is welcome and essential. This may take the form of:

(a)   days out from home on tours or picnics or in day centres.

(b)   relief for the attendants by the use of relief home helps or visiting attendants.

(c)   holidays for the disabled person at specially organized centres.

(d)   Admission of the patient to an institution to enable the relatives to go on regular holidays.

If the patient's relatives and attendants are to continue gladly to supply physical care, mental stimulation and affection, they must have the opportunity to develop outside interests and activities. Nurses in hospital have days off; attending relatives have similar needs!

Recent legislation in the United Kingdom

The most far-reaching government legislation for the disabled person in the United Kingdom is the Chronically Sick and Disabled Persons Act 1970. This makes the local authority responsible for many facets of management of disabled persons within its boundary. This is the first time that such comprehensive legislation has existed. A summary of their functions is as follows:

1   Establishing the number and needs of disabled people.

2   Ensuring that the disabled and their families are fully aware of the help which is available to them and how it may be obtained.

3   Providing comprehensive help such as:

(a)   A telephone specially adapted to the needs of the individual

(b)   Meals, served either at home or in a special centre

(c)   Facilities for taking holidays

(d)   Assistance in carrying out adaptations to the home

(e)   Travelling facilities
(f)   Educational opportunities
(g)   Recreational facilities
(h)   Radio, television, library or similar recreational facilities
(i)   Practical assistance in organizing and running the household.
4   Practical specially provided for the public use of disabled persons.

(a)   Sign-posting to special facilities provided for the disabled, (see Fig. 13.1).

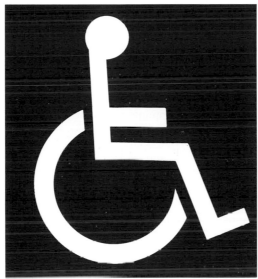

Fig. 13.1.   The universal disabled persons symbol.

(b)   Supplying special access via ramps or level places to public lavatories, parking places, libraries, swimming pools and similar places (Fig 6.10).

(c)   Supplying comprehensive sanitary conveniences especially for the disabled.

All of these are supervised by special Advisory Committees which consist of people with special knowledge of the needs of the disabled.

Similar legislation exists or is evolving in most countries of the world but often the vigor with which the laws are executed is inadequate or negative.

Social security in the United Kingdom

The United Kingdom has had a comprehensive social security system for many years and this affects the paralysed and disabled person. Such a system means that inability to go out to employment does not result in starvation and severe deprivation.

Such provisions are constantly undergoing change and it is unwise to record precise details in a textbook. It is always necessary to find out the current provisions under social security from the free leaflets and booklets supplied by the Department of Health and Social Secutiry.

Examples of these are:

(a)   FAMILY ALLOWANCES

Cash payments for families with more than one child under school leaving age.

(b)   FAMILY INCOMES SUPPLEMENT

This is a benefit available to those families whose normal gross weekly income is low. The rate of supplement equals one half of the difference between the family's normal gross income and an amount decided by Parliament and modified from time to time. Additionally the family does not pay prescription charges for drugs supplied under the National Health Service, dental charges or optical charges. Children at school are allowed free meals and expectant mothers and children under five years are given free welfare foods and milk.

(c)   SUPPLEMENTARY BENEFITS

These supplement the income of people who are not in full employment and whose total income is not enough to meet their needs. Additionally there is an allowance for rent and an allowance for special expenses such as an invalid diet, extra heating, because of age or disability and domestic help. These benefits are paid as a right but it is often difficult to convince aged and needy people that they are not receiving charity. Travelling expenses for visits to hospital by patients attending for treatment or consultation, are paid for by the state.

(d)   ATTENDANCE ALLOWANCE

This is a tax-free allowance to severely disabled persons who for the past six months, at least, are either so physically or mentally disabled that he requires help from another person frequently during the day and repeatedly during the night.

(e)   SICKNESS BENEFIT

This is the allowance paid to all who have contributed to the National

Insurance scheme during employment or self-employment, for the first twenty-eight weeks of any illness.

(f)   INVALIDITY BENEFITS

Replaces sickness benefits after the twenty-eight weeks of illness and is given to people who become chronically ill whilst they still have a large part of their normal working lives ahead of them. The amount given is related to the age or capacity; the younger the patient the larger the allowance.

(g)   INJURY AND DISABLEMENT BENEFITS

These are payments to people injured at work or who contract an industrial disease and are subsequently unable to work.

Conclusions

In helping the chronically disabled it is important not to overprotect and destroy the patient's own efforts and initiative. It is important to know what the patient and his or her relatives can be expected to do. This is where outside aid is essential. Both the patients and relatives must learn to accept what cannot be changed but to strive for change and improvement where this is possible.

Glossary

Abduction: Movement of a limb away from the midline of the body.

Adduction: Movement of a limb towards the midline of the body.

Afferent: Towards the centre. Relevant to nerves and blood vessels.

Agnosia: Disturbance in recognition of sensory impression.

Aneurysm: Abnormal dilatation of an artery.

Ankylosis: The condition in which a joint is stiffened by either fibrous tissue or bony fusion.

Anoxia: Absence of oxygen.

Aphasia: Inability to speak.

Approximate: To bring together two ends.

Apraxia: Inability to perform some purposive movements.

Arteriosclerosis: Degeneration of an artery with loss of flexibility of its walls.

Arthrogryposis: Flexure of a joint. Congenital generalized stiffness of the joints of the arms and legs.

Ataxia: A condition in which voluntary movements are not properly organised. Lack of co-ordination.

Athetosis: A condition in which there are involuntary, useless, disordered movements.

Avulsion: Forcible separation of two parts.

Axillary: Pertaining to the armpit.

Catheterization: Passage of fluids through an instrument; most commonly urine from the bladder.

Cavus: The longitudinal arch of the foot becomes abnormally high.

Cervical: Pertaining to the neck.

Chemotherapy: Healing by the use of chemicals.

Clonus: A turmoil or tumult. Reflex irregular contraction of muscles.

Conservative Treatment: Aiming at preservation or repair.

Contracture: Fixed contraction due to fibrous tissue formation.

Contusion: Stagnant blood in soft tissue after an injury. A bruise.

Cubitus: Pertaining to the elbow joint

Cutaneous: Pertaining to the skin.

Cyst: A cavity or space.

Decubitus: Lying down. Relevant to a sore caused by the pressure of the weight of the body.

Deformity: Abnormality affecting posture.

Degeneration: Progressive deterioration.

Denervation: Deprivation of nerve supply.

Dermatome: Area of skin innervated by a single spinal nerve.

Devitalised: Deprived of a blood supply.

Diplopia: Double vision.

Disseminated: Scattered throughout; in this example, the nervous system.

Drop-Foot: Deformity in which the forefoot hangs down and cannot be raised.

Dysarthria: Impairment of speech.

Dystrophy: Abnormal growth.

Efferent: From the centre to the periphery.

Elective Surgery: A surgical procedure performed at the convenience of the patient and the surgeon.

Elongation: To increase the length of a bone or tendon.

Equinus: A deformity in which the foot points downwards and the patient walks on the heads of the metatarsal bones.

Erosion: Degenerative destruction.

Extracerebral: Outside, but relevant to, the cerebrum.

Extradural: Exterior to the dura mater.

Extrinsic: External. From without.

Fistula: An abnormal passage connecting one epithelial surface with another.

Flaccidity: Lacking rigidity; floppy.

Gliosis: An increase in the supporting tissue of nervous tissue.

Hemianaesthesia: Anaesthesia of one side only.

Hemianopia: Loss of sight in one half of the visual field.

Hemiplegia: Paralysis of one side of the body.

Herpes: Vesicular eruption caused by infection.

Horner's Syndrome: One-sided pupil contraction, ptosis and vasodilation of the cheek with absence of sweating.

Hydrocephalus: Swelling of the head in young children or infants caused by raised intracranial pressure.

Hyperflexion: Excessive flexion; greater than is normal.

Imbalance: Lack of balance; pertaining to muscle contraction at joints.

Incontinence: Absence of control over the passing of urine and faeces.

Intracerebral: Within the cerebrum.

Intradural: Within the dura mater.

Intrinsic: Inherent to a part.

Ischaemia: An inadequate or deficient blood supply to part because of obstruction of blood-vessels.

Kyphosis: Forward curvature of the spine.

Laminectomy: Excision of part of the lamina of the vertebra to gain access to the neural canal or increase the opening for the pathway of a spinal nerve.

Lateral: On the side; away from the mid line.

Lesion: Injury or pathological change in the structure or function of a part of the body.

Lordosis: Spinal curvature which is anteriorly convex.

Meningitis: Inflammation of the meninges due to infection.

Metatarsalgia: Pain in the part of the foot in the metatarsal region.

Motor Neurone: Neurones passing out from a nerve centre conveying an order of motion.

Movements, Active: Movements which are the result of a patient's own muscular activity.

Movements, Passive: Movements applied to joints, by a physiotherapist or nurse, without muscular effort on the part of the patient.

Myasthenia: Loss of power in muscle groups.

Myelitis: Inflammation of the spinal cord.

Myelography: Radiography of the spinal-cord.

Myelomeningocoele: A pouch of meninges containing nervous tissue and cerebrospinal fluid the result of a defect in the spine of an infant.

Myopathy: Any disease of a muscle.

Myositis: Inflammation of muscle.

Neurapraxia: Temporary block to nerve conduction.

Neuroglioma: A tumour of the special connective tissue of the nervous system.

Neuroma: A tumour of a nerve:

Neuromuscular: Pertaining both to nerve and muscle.

Neuropathy: With a weak or absent nerve organisation.

Neurotmesis: Severance or severe crushing of a nerve trunk.

Oliguria: Severe diminution of the quantity of urine excreted.

Otorrhoea: A discharge from the ear.

Paralysis: A faulty or absent nerve supply.

Paraplegia: Paralysis affecting the lower half of the body.

Paresis: Partial paralysis.

Periphery: Away from the centre; towards the surface or circumference.

Pes: Pertaining to the foot.

Polymyositis: Inflammation resulting in weakening and wasting of muscles.

Plantigrade: The normal position of the foot in relation to tibia and fibula, neither raised or lowered, nor everted or inverted.

Plexus: A grouping or cluster of nerve trunks.

Posterior: The dorsal surface of the body or part of the body. The opposite surface to the anterior.

Posture: The position of the body.

Prone: Lying with the front of the body downwards.

Prophylaxis: Tending to prevent disease.

Prosthesis: An apparatus used to replace an absent limb, part of a limb, or an organ.

Protoplasm: The living substance which forms the main part of the tissue-cells of the body.

Proximal: Nearest to the centre, when applied to a limb.

Pseudohypertrophic: A false increase in size.

Pyelonephritis: Inflammation of the kidney and its pelvis.

Rhinorrhoea: Discharge from the nose.

Sclerosis: Hardening.

Scoliosis: The deformity of the spine which exists when the spine is curved to the side.

Sensory: Afferent. Carrying information into the central nervous system.

Skeletal: Pertaining to the skeleton.

Spasm: Involuntary contraction of muscle tissue

Spasticity: Imperfect voluntary control of muscles with stiff jerking movements.

Spina Bifida: Failure of fusion of one or more vertebral arches resulting in a congenital malformation.

Stability: Steadiness, firmness.

Stabilization: Fixation of a paralysed joint to support the weight of the body, or limb, in a steady posture.

Stasis: Arrest of movement of body fluids or intestinal contents.

Supine: Lying horizontal with the anterior surface of the body uppermost. Also with the palm of the hand upwards when pertaining to the forearm.

Syringo-Myelia: Progressive disease in which the brain stem and spinal cord degenerate.

Talipes: Deformities in which the tarsal-joints are involved.

Tetraplegia: Paralysis affecting all four limbs.

Thrombosis: Coagulation of the blood within the circulatory system.

Thrombus: A clot of blood within the circulatory system.

Tic: Twitching of the muscles, usually of face and neck.

Traction: The application of a pulling force to a limb to overcome muscle spasm.

Transplantation: Surgical transfer of tissue from one part of the body to another.

Trauma: A wound or injury.

Tumour: A swelling or enlargement which is abnormal.

Unilateral: Affecting one side only.

Valgus: Divergence of the part indicated away from the mid-line of the body.

Varus: Bent. A term applied to bow-legs or club-feet.

INDEX

DATE DUE
